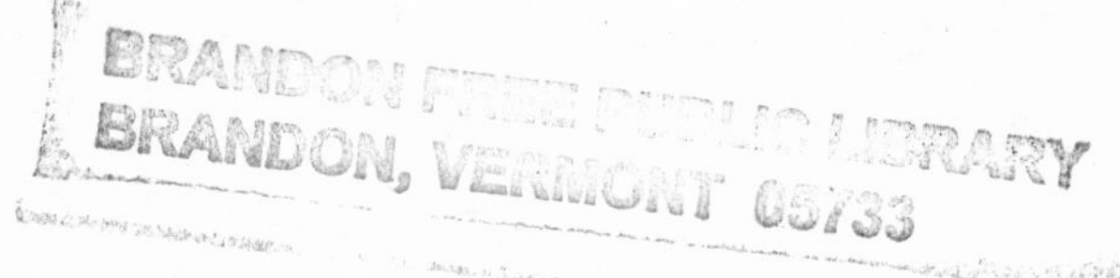

The Back Almanac

First printing 1992

Distributed to the book trade by:
Ten Speed Press
P.O. Box 7123
Berkeley, CA 94707

Cover Design by Ken Scott
Book Design & Production by Fifth Street Design, Berkeley, California
Edited by Judy Berman, Blair Carroll, Pamela Valdés
Production by J.C. Wright
Illustrations by Ginger Beringer, Thos Chapman, Giselle Kuster, Mina Reimer

To contact the publishers, please write to:
Lanier Publishing International, Ltd.
P.O. Box 20429
Oakland, CA 94620

Library of Congress Cataloging-in-Publication Data

The Back Almanac / by the editors of Lanier Publishing
p. cm.
Includes bibliographical references and index.
ISBN 0-89815-508-8
1. Backache – Popular works. I. Lanier Publishing.
RD771.B217B29 1992
617.5'64 – dc20 92-25976
CIP

Printed in the United States of America on recycled paper.
1 2 3 4 5 – 96 95 94 93 92

TABLE OF CONTENTS

Acknowledgments

Many thanks to the following people who shared their time and expertise with us in the making of this book:

Sarah Key for sharing with us her unique voice and perspective; Dr. William Meeker and Dr. Thomas Milus for their written contribution; Karen Perlroth for her article and her willingness to work with us to make this book a success; Dr. Mary Pullig Schatz for her written contribution and Donald Moyer and Linda Cogozzo of Rodmell Press for making her work available to us; Jennifer Atkins for her written contribution; Ellen Best Lagerwerff for providing us with drawings from her book *Houding – Gezondheid – Elegance*; Dierdre Frank, Dr. Hubert Rosomoff and Lawrence Galton for their written contributions; Artists Ginger Beringer, Thos Chapman and Mina Reimer; Carol Berman, RPA, for her research assistance and patience.

Special thanks to: Dr. David I. Greenly, MD, FACEP, Medical Director of Emergency Services at Alta Bates-Herrick Hospital, for his written contribution as well as his professional review of the chapters *The First 48 Hours, Disaster First Aid,* and *Diagnostic Tests*; Dr. Arthur Berman, MD, Director of Medicine at Lawrence Hospital, Assistant Clinical Professor at Albert Einstein College of Medicine and Adjunct Attending Physician at Montefiore Medical Center for his professional review of the chapters *The Medical Doctor's Visit, Causes of Back Pain,* and *Drug Therapy,* his many helpful suggestions and his overall support of the project.

This book cannot and does not offer medical advice. We cannot and do not endorse any of the treatment modes described in the book, but provide them only to inform the reader of the many modes of treatment available. We urge that you seek advice from a qualified health care provider for any back problem you may have. Neither the publisher nor any of the authors published in the book may be held liable for any injury, loss, or damage sustained by anyone who relies on the information contained in the book.

INTRODUCTION

What are you doing as you read this? Are you standing in a bookstore leaning one shoulder against the bookshelves? Or are you sitting with your legs crossed? Maybe you're curled up on a soft comfortable sofa or maybe you're sitting in a desk chair, leaning over your desk. If you were not aware of your posture at this moment, you are not alone. Most Americans have very little idea of the effect of their everyday movements on their health. But perhaps you're lying in bed with a backache, painfully aware of your posture. If so, then you're one of those 75-80 million Americans, one of the 4 out of 5 that everyone's talking about who suffer back pain at some point in their lives.

The numbers are pretty clear – Most people in the United States know what it's like to feel back pain. The US Department of Health and Human Services reported that 19 million doctor visits are made for back pain annually, with 8 million new cases every year. The FDA Consumer reported that, "on any given day, 6.5 million Americans are under some sort of treatment for low back pain." Back pain is topped only by sore throats as America's most common ailment. Figures for the cost of backaches in treatment, lost wages, and workman's compensation range from $16 to $60 Billion a year!

But what most people don't know is that it's not only heavy lifting that causes back pain. More often it's the way you sit, stand, read, eat, day in and day out. If you bend at the waist to pick up a piece of clothing, sit at a desk for hours without standing and stretching, stand with your back arched because of a pot belly, slump over your dinner because you're tired from working all day, then you're setting yourself up for an attack of back pain. And if your back says no once, chances are four times more likely that it will happen again.

But whether you're in bed with your first or fiftieth attack, or whether you've never had a back problem in your life, it's not too early or too late to think about taking better care of your back. Research has shown that the best insurance against back trouble is exercising and strengthening the muscles which support the spine. And you can begin to do that even from the bed where you're recovering from back surgery.

In this book you'll find a collection of different approaches to back care, and what to expect from different kinds of health care professionals and their treatments, all prepared to help you to select your own best option. Everyone's back is different, and everyone's pain is different. The important thing is to ask questions, do research, and find the assistance that YOU need to help YOU take better care of yourself for life.

Please be aware that the information provided here does not constitute medical advice. We cannot and do not endorse any of the treatment modes described in the book, but provide them only to inform you of the many modes of treatment available. If you have any concerns about your condition, we urge you to seek advice from a qualified health care provider. The decisions you make concerning your health care are your own responsibility. We are not liable for any injury, loss or damage sustained by someone relying on the information contained in the book.

"Although men and women are affected with low back pain with approximately equal frequency, work-related injuries for which compensation is received are much more common in men. The occupation with the highest rate of compensable back injuries is truck driving. Material handlers have been found to be at the next highest risk. High rates of compensable back injury are also present among nurses and nursing aides who have to perform many of the same types of tasks as those handling heavy objects in industry."

– United States Department of Health and Human Services, *Report on Low Back Pain*

DANGER SIGNALS

See a doctor immediately:

1. If the pain you're experiencing is profoundly agonizing (or wakes you up at night).
2. You have a loss of bladder or bowel control, high fever or sore throat.
3. Severe abdominal pain.
4. Very dark or bloody stools or vomitus.
5. Severe menstrual pain or heavy vaginal bleeding
6. A severe backache that persists more than 3 days, after you've taken aspirin or other pain reliever and had complete, horizontal, bedrest.
7. Shooting pain down your arm or leg, numbness or muscle weakness.
8. Back pain in a child or elderly person.

"Long-distance driving, cigarette smoking, coughing, prolonged standing, prolonged sitting without changing position, lifting heavy objects, twisting, performing sudden physical efforts, and working with vibrating tools may all predispose to LBP [Low Back Pain]."
– Abital Fast, MD

It is extremely important to remember that just because you've had back pain before, it doesn't mean that your current backache is the same. Back pain can be caused by everything from muscle strain to ulcers to ovarian tumors. If you are feeling at all uncertain, check with your physician. If you see your doctor, and your back pain is not responding to the recommended treatment, consider seeing another doctor in a different field of specialization. Different specialists, including and sometimes especially the best in their field, are trained to look for, and therefore to find different things. The neurologist, for example, probably won't perform a pelvic exam and may or may not consider such sources

§ *Get a reaching tool. There are two on the market:*

– Matley Reaching Aid, that has a magnetic tip and a positive grip controlled by your hand pressure. It can pick up clothes off the floor, pins, pens, or any lightweight object lying around the floor, except the family pet and hard plastic cases (like cassette cases). Even if you don't use it all the time, it's great for getting to items that have slipped behind the bookcase or couch.

– The second is an EZ Reacher for kitchen or workshop use. It has large rubber cups that can pick up a coin or a can of soup – anything that fits between the two rubber gripping tongs and weighs less than a couple of pounds. The grip locks in place, so you don't have to squeeze it continuously. (See Back Designs in the Catalog section)

of back pain. Remember that, although as many as 90% of back pain episodes are caused by muscle strain, back pain can be indicative of serious health problems. Delayed diagnosis and delayed treatment can be life threatening. Don't ignore the danger signals.

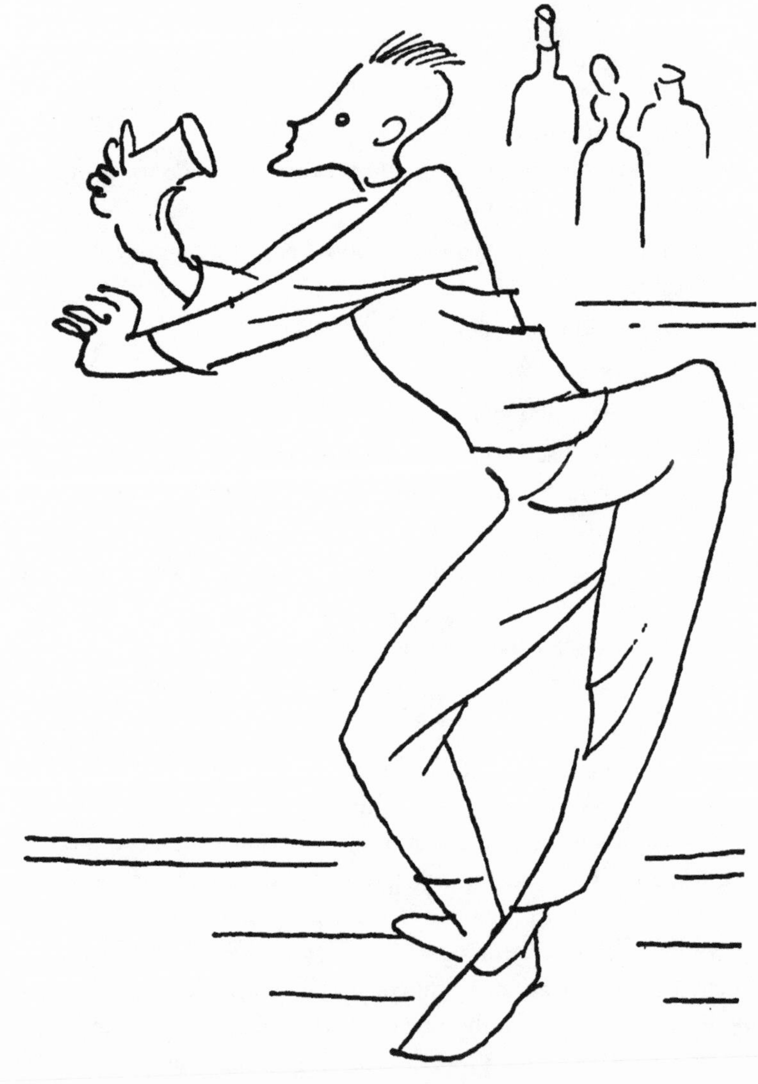

THE FIRST 48 HOURS

What To Do If Your Back Just Went "Out"

1. Immediately STOP whatever you are doing.
2. Make an ice pack. Lie down and put the ice pack on the injured portion of your back for 20 minutes every 2-3 hours (for the first 48 hours, except while sleeping). Always put a thin layer like a tea towel between your skin and the ice pack. Try using a large size bag of frozen peas that can conform to the area. (You can refreeze and use them for many treatments, but do not use them for eating.) If the problem is in a very localized spot, a can of frozen fruit juice may be just right.

   NOTE: Ice reduces swelling, and can help break the pain-muscle spasm syndrome. If ice causes further discomfort, do not use. Or try alternating with heat, using ice for 20 minutes and then heat.
3. Take 500-650 mg. acetominophen (Tylenol) tablets or 400 mg. of ibuprofen (Advil/Motrin) immediately.
4. Remain in bed except to use the bathroom! Get help for meal making and other tasks. If you absolutely have no one else, get simple meals while you are up. Your body needs a chance to heal and lying down is the best position to accomplish this. Most severe muscle strains and sprains will respond to this treatment within 48 hours. After 48 hours switch to heat treatments for 20 minutes, 2 to 3 times daily. Get out of bed, but take it easy: no prolonged sitting, no sudden movements.
5. If your back is not feeling much better, see a doctor.

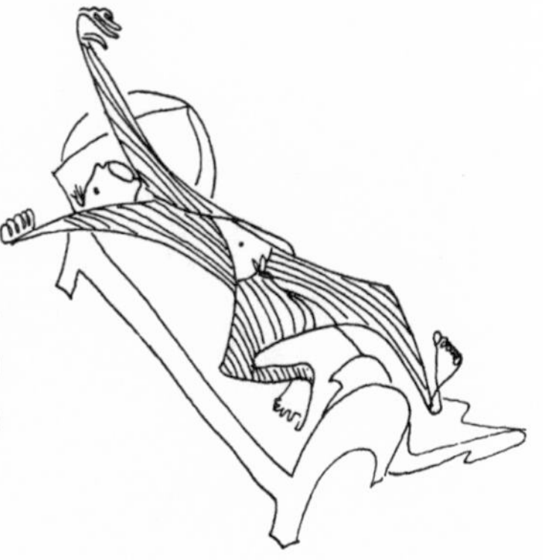

"Proper bed rest and physical therapy can put 80% of lower back sufferers back on their feet in less than a week."
— Ridley Pearson

NOTE: This emergency treatment is also useful for slipped discs.

❍ ASPIRIN TIPS

Aspirin is a genuine miracle drug, and can be very helpful due to its pain relieving and anti-inflammatory action. However, aspirin increases bleeding time. If you have "pulled your back" or "strained" a muscle, there will be small capillary bleeding in the muscle which will be increased with aspirin. Aspirin is also associated with gastro-intestinal problems, like ulcers and bleeding.

If you have a history of gastric ulcers, avoid aspirin and use acetominophen (Tylenol). Another non-steroidal anti-inflammatory drug (NSAID) which is milder than aspirin is ibuprofen (Motrin, Advil). Be careful: do not take ibuprofen if you have had a severe reaction to aspirin. Although these do not contain aspirin, cross-reactions may occur. Ask your doctor which one would be the best for you, based on your health history. Even ibuprofen can create and aggravate gastrointestinal disorders. There is a drug available (misoprostol or Cytotec) that has been found to help with the gastrointestinal symptoms associated with NSAIDs like aspirin and ibuprofen, but be aware that this drug has side effects of its own.

Some people find pain relievers difficult to take. The following tips may make it easier:

- *Try the mildest pain reliever first.*
- *Take the pain reliever with food and plenty of fluid.*
- *If you prefer aspirin, use buffered or coated aspirin (the most effectively buffered aspirin is Alka-Seltzer).*
- *If this doesn't work, try chasing the aspirin with peptol bismol or an antacid, (but be aware that antacids can also be harmful if overused).*

"With the arms and upper part of the spine acting as levers on the bottom of your back, the force on your discs can equal 2000 to 3000 pounds per square inch. Also, the lower back muscles are tremendously powerful and can produce huge compressive forces on the discs."

– William Southmayd, MD, *Sports Health*

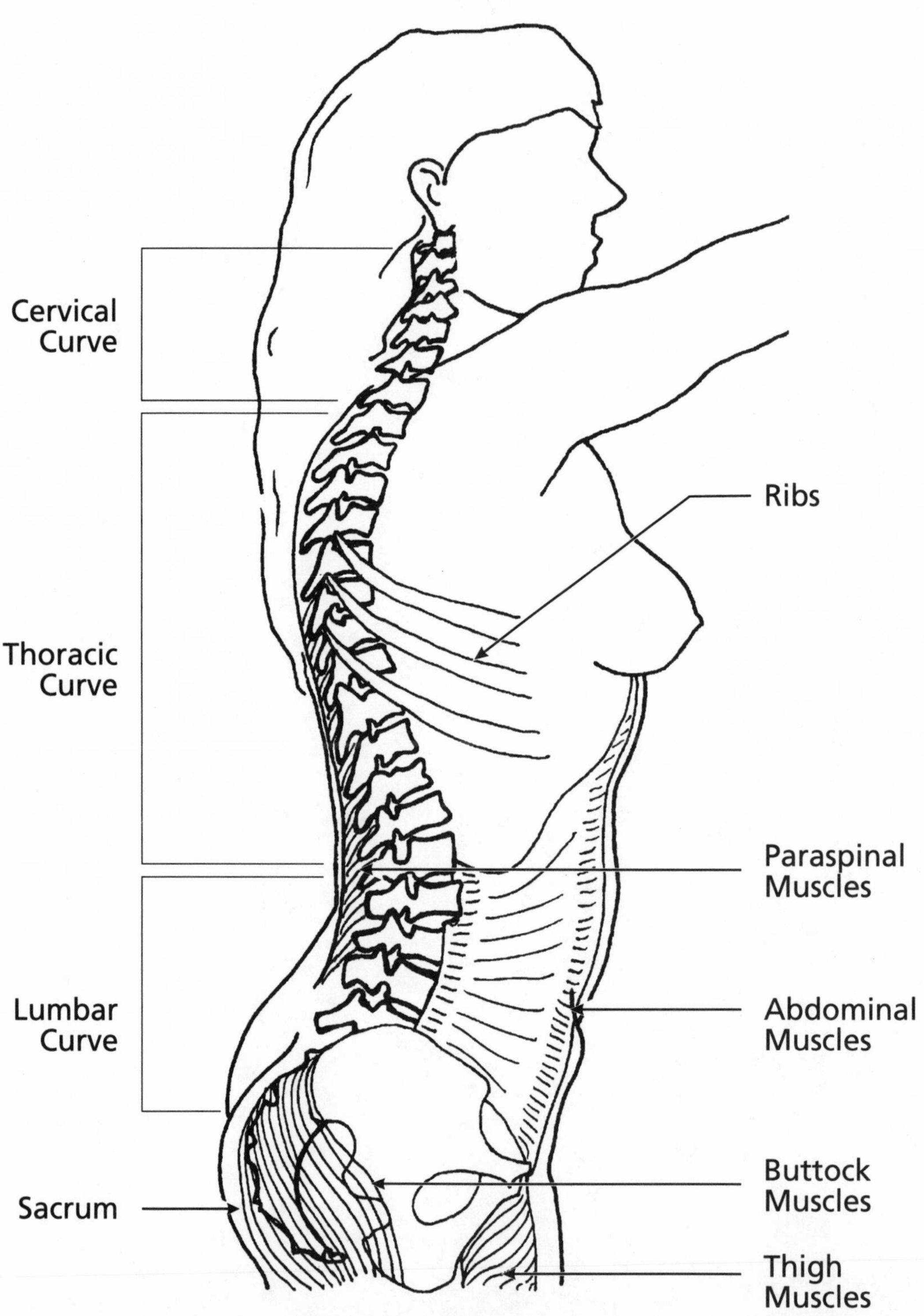
Cervical
Curve
Thoracic
Curve
Lumbar
Curve
Sacrum
Ribs
Paraspinal
Muscles
Abdominal
Muscles
Buttock
Muscles
Thigh
Muscles

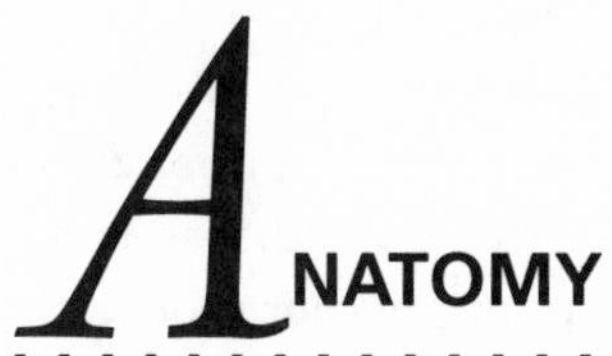

NATOMY

Understanding Your Back

Excerpted from Back Care Basics: A Doctor's Gentle Yoga Program for Back and Neck Pain Relief, *by Mary Pullig Schatz, M.D.*

To heal your back, you must understand it. Back pain results from a complex combination of factors, including posture, congenital disorders, and attitudes toward life. Viewing your pain as an illness isolated from the rest of your life may keep you from changing habits that may be perpetuating it.

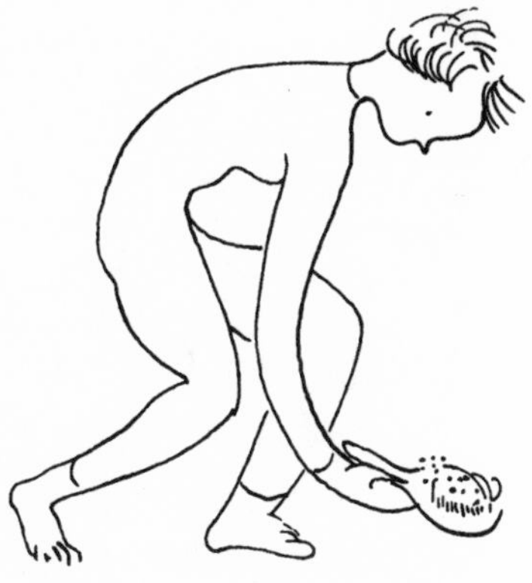

Back problems do not occur in a vacuum. The spine is not an isolated body part. For a therapeutic approach to chronic back or neck strain to succeed, the spine must be seen as an integral component of a whole human being.

Your whole body affects your back. The mechanical function of your spine affects and is affected by the alignment, flexibility, and strength of many parts of your body, including:

- *Foot, knee, and leg alignment*
- *Muscle strength of legs, buttocks, back, and abdominal wall*
- *Abdominal protrusion (as with a beer belly or pregnancy)*
- *Hip flexibility*
- *The position of the pelvis (tilted forward, back, or to either side)*
- *The shape and flexibility of the lumbar (lower back) spinal curve*
- *The shape and flexibility of the thoracic (upper back) spinal curve*

- *Shoulder carriage and the mobility of the arms at the shoulder joints*
- *The shape of the cervical (neck) spinal curve*
- *The position of the head in relation to the shoulders*

§ *When standing for long periods of time put one foot up a step (on a small box, or the rung of a chair). About the height of two phone books. This will take the pressure off the lower back. There is a good reason why a metal bar runs along the bottom of most bars.*

For example, if your shoulder joints can't move freely, you will compensate by overarching your lower back when you reach overhead. Misalignments of your feet, knees, and legs (for example, pigeon toes, flat feet, and leg-length differences) are transferred upward, distorting your pelvis and spine. If your head is held forward of your shoulders, the muscles of your neck and upper back must overwork, creating neck pain and tension headaches.

To be effective, back care must not be confined to exercise time, but incorporated into a new way of life. An hour of therapeutic exercise can't make up for twenty hours of destructive movements.

SPINAL ANATOMY AND FUNCTION

To begin to understand the sources of your particular back problem, it helps to understand the anatomy of the spine.

The spine is a series of 24 intricately interlocking spool-shaped bones called *vertebrae,* supported by a complex system of muscles and ligaments. The hollow spinal canal, formed by the bony arches protruding from the back of each vertebra, protects the nerve tissue of the spinal cord.

The arms, legs, and chest all attach to the spine, via the shoulder girdle, pelvis, and ribs. The weight of the head is perched on the end of the spine. Therefore, the spine affects and is affected by every movement your body makes. For example, if the head is not properly balanced, the natural curve of the neck becomes distorted. If the arms or legs don't have a full range of motion, the spine must compensate by extra bending and twisting. Conversely, if the spine is not functioning properly, the arms, legs and head can't move freely either. And without proper spinal alignment, the internal organs will be compressed.

The natural curves of the spine are vitally important, allowing it to act as a shock absorber during the jolts of walking, running, and sitting in a moving vehicle. The curves give the spine a strength and resilience many times that of a straight and rigid column. As an analogy, consider the difference in shock-absorbing capacity between a metal spring and a rigid pole. If you slam the end of a pole onto a hard surface, you will feel an uncomfortable jarring impact. But if you do the same thing with a coiled spring of the same material, the force will be absorbed by the spring, rather than transmitted to your body.

Viewed from the side, the curves of the spine are:

- *Cervical (neck): convex in front*
- *Thoracic (upper back): convex behind*
- *Lumbar (lower back): convex in front*

These normal curves lie in the front-to-back plane of the body. Too much or too little curve in any of these areas can lead to dysfunction.

VERTEBRAE

The lumbar vertebrae are massive (approximately two inches in diameter), reflecting their weight-bearing role. The cervical vertebrae are smaller, since they must support only the head. The bodies of the vertebrae are solid, roughly cylindrical blocks of bone that stack on one another, separated by the intervertebral discs. To the rear of each vertebral body, bony projections extend back from each side to form the neural arches that make up the spinal canal, which protects the spinal cord. The muscles that bend and rotate the spine are attached to these bony projections (which are called the spinous and transverse processes).

§ *Ask for help if the task is too great: Split lifting jobs. If you have 200 seed bags to move, space the labor over time. Lifting when you're fatigued leads to back strain.*

Branching off of each of the transverse processes are flat surfaces called facets, which are similar to the facets of a cut gem. The facets of one vertebra form joints (facet joints) with the facets of the vertebrae above and below. The slant of the facet surfaces determines the directions the vertebrae can move. Back or neck pain identical to that caused by a herniated intervertebral disc can be caused by abnormalities (such as arthritis) in the facet joints.

INTERVERTEBRAL DISCS

Discs are thick pads of cartilage that separate adjacent vertebrae. Together, they make up one-fourth of the length of the vertebral column. The discs serve as shock absorbers and allow greater motion between the vertebrae than would be possible if the bones were in direct contact with each other. Most important, they distribute weight over a large surface when the spine bends. When discs degenerate, this weight becomes concentrated on the edges of the vertebrae, resulting in bone spurs.

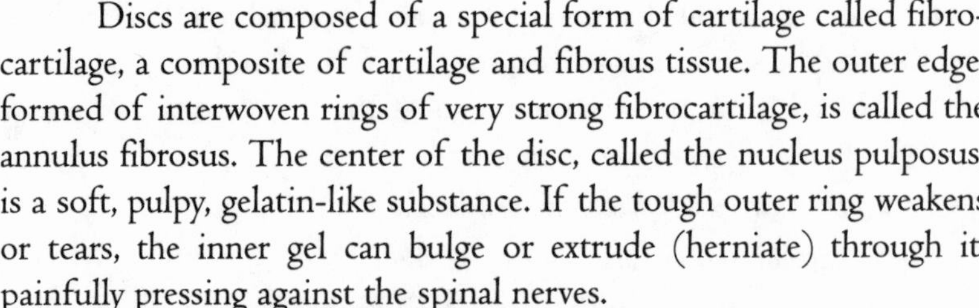

Discs are composed of a special form of cartilage called fibrocartilage, a composite of cartilage and fibrous tissue. The outer edge, formed of interwoven rings of very strong fibrocartilage, is called the annulus fibrosus. The center of the disc, called the nucleus pulposus, is a soft, pulpy, gelatin-like substance. If the tough outer ring weakens or tears, the inner gel can bulge or extrude (herniate) through it, painfully pressing against the spinal nerves.

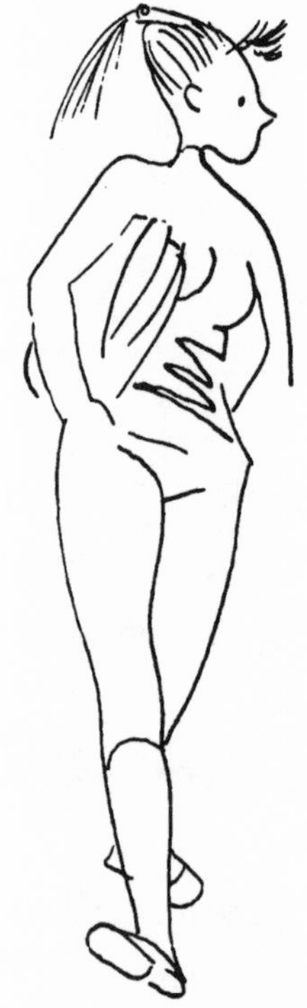

The disc acquires its nourishment through the fluid-attracting and fluid-absorbing qualities of the gel-like nucleus pulposus. With no blood supply of its own, the disc is dependent on sponge action for attracting and absorbing nutrients from adjacent tissues. During nonweight-bearing rest, the discs expand as they soak up fluid, increasing the length of the spine by as much as one inch overnight. In weight-bearing activity, this fluid is squeezed back into the adjacent soft tissues and vertebrae, to be replaced by fresh fluid during the next rest period. If these normal healing mechanisms are inhibited by poor posture and loss of flexibility, the discs become thin, brittle, and easily injured. This condition, called degenerative disc disease, can lead to bulging or herniated discs.

❍ SPINAL CORD AND NERVE ROOTS

Literally an extension of the brain, the spinal cord is a bundle of nerves that travels down through the spinal canal, which is formed by a series of arches in the vertebrae (the neural arches, discussed earlier). When a nerve branches off of the cord, it exits the spinal column via an intervertebral foramen (a hole between two vertebrae). At this exit point, the nerve is vulnerable to compression by a bulging or herniated intervertebral disc.

❍ SACRUM AND PELVIS

The pelvis is a funnel-shaped group of relatively flat bones, higher in the back than in the front. Because the joints between the bones of the pelvis allow very little motion, the pelvis effectively functions as a single bone. The end of the spinal column (the tailbone and the flat, triangular bone called the sacrum, which is formed by the fusion of the last five vertebrae) forms part of the back wall of the pelvis, and the upper ends of the thigh bones insert into sockets in its side walls. Thus, the pelvis joins the spine to the legs.

Because the end of the spine (the sacrum) forms part of the pelvic funnel, the position of the pelvis has profound effects on the lumbar curve. You can experience this connection by performing this simple exercise: Sit on a firm chair with a flat seat. Tilt your pelvis forward so your navel moves forward toward your knees and your tailbone moves up and back. With your hands on your back, feel how this motion increases the lumbar curve to a more swaybacked position. Now tilt your pelvis backward by tucking your tailbone and moving your navel toward your spine. Notice how your lumbar spine flattens.

§ Don't sit in bed – unless you think strongly about back support. Sitting in bed with your feet horizontally out in front of you with poor or non-existent back support doesn't seem threatening, but can create problems over time.

❍ MUSCLES THAT ACT ON THE SPINE

The bony structures of the spine and pelvis are supported and moved by many different muscles, whose condition can profoundly affect the state of your lower back. If any of these muscles are tight or weak, they can create or worsen back pain.

Running parallel to your spine are the paraspinal muscles, deep muscles of the back that function as guy wires to support the spine in the upright position. (To feel the paraspinal, put your hand on your back at waist level. The slight bulges you feel on either side of the spine are formed by the paraspinal muscles.) The paraspinals rotate the spine, bend it backward and sideways, and influence posture by helping create and maintain the proper spinal curves. If the paraspinals are too tight, they contribute to a swayback. If they are too stretched out, they contribute to a flat back. If they are overworked, they can go into painful spasms.

The lower back is also significantly influenced by three sets of muscles that attach to the pelvis or the lumbar vertebrae: the hip flexors (which raise the thigh toward the chest), the abdominals, and the hamstrings (the long muscles on the back of the thigh). By altering the forward or backward tilt of the pelvis, these muscles can increase or decrease the lumbar curve. For example, because the hip flexors attach to the front of the pelvis, tight hip flexors will tilt the pelvis forward, creating a swayback. Tight hamstrings will tilt the pelvis backward, creating a flat back. Weak abdominal muscles will allow the pelvis to drop forward and will fail to support the lumbar spine from the front.

❍ YOUR NECK AND YOUR BACK

Since it is actually a part of the spine, your neck can be affected by many of the same conditions that affect your back, including muscle strain, degenerative disc disease, and arthritis. When they are chronically stressed, the intervertebral discs in the neck can also bulge or herniate. A herniated cervical disc can cause pain, weakness, or numbness in the shoulder, arm, or hand.

❍ JOINTS AND MUSCLES

Each of your joints is controlled by at least two sets of muscles: the flexors, which bend the joint, and the extensors, which straighten it. In addition, a number of joints have rotator muscles that twist, turn, or rotate the bones. Good posture can exist only when the flexors, extensors, and rotators are in proper balance, allowing each joint to function efficiently. In a well-balanced joint, the cartilage surfaces at the ends of the bones move against each other in a way that promotes orderly repair of the joint tissues.

But often, the muscles acting upon a joint are out of balance. For example, the flexors may be tighter and shorter than the extensors, so that the joint cannot be fully straightened; or the muscles that rotate the joint in one direction may be stronger than those that rotate it the other way. These unequal forces make the joint weaker and more vulnerable. Parts of the bone surfaces bear more weight than they should. By altering the normal regenerative processes that keep joints healthy, this imbalance can cause pain and arthritis.

Many people with back or neck pain suffer from an imbalance of the flexors, extensors, and rotators of the spine, arms and legs. With an intelligent program of stretching and strengthening, like yoga, for example, the muscle groups can be brought back into balance.

§ *Take your time. There is more of a chance you will injure your muscles when you're not thinking about how you are using them.*

About the Author:

Mary Pullig Schatz, M.D., is a pathologist and certified Iyengar-style yoga teacher. She practices medicine and yoga in Nashville, Tennessee, where she is Medical Staff President at Centennial Medical Center. She is a regular contributor to the "Exercise Adviser" column for *The Physician and Sportsmedicine* and is the author of *Back Care Basics: A Doctor's Gentle Yoga Program for Back and Neck Pain Relief* (Rodmell Press, 1992). Dr. Schatz teaches Back and Neck Care Basics Seminars℠ throughout the United States.

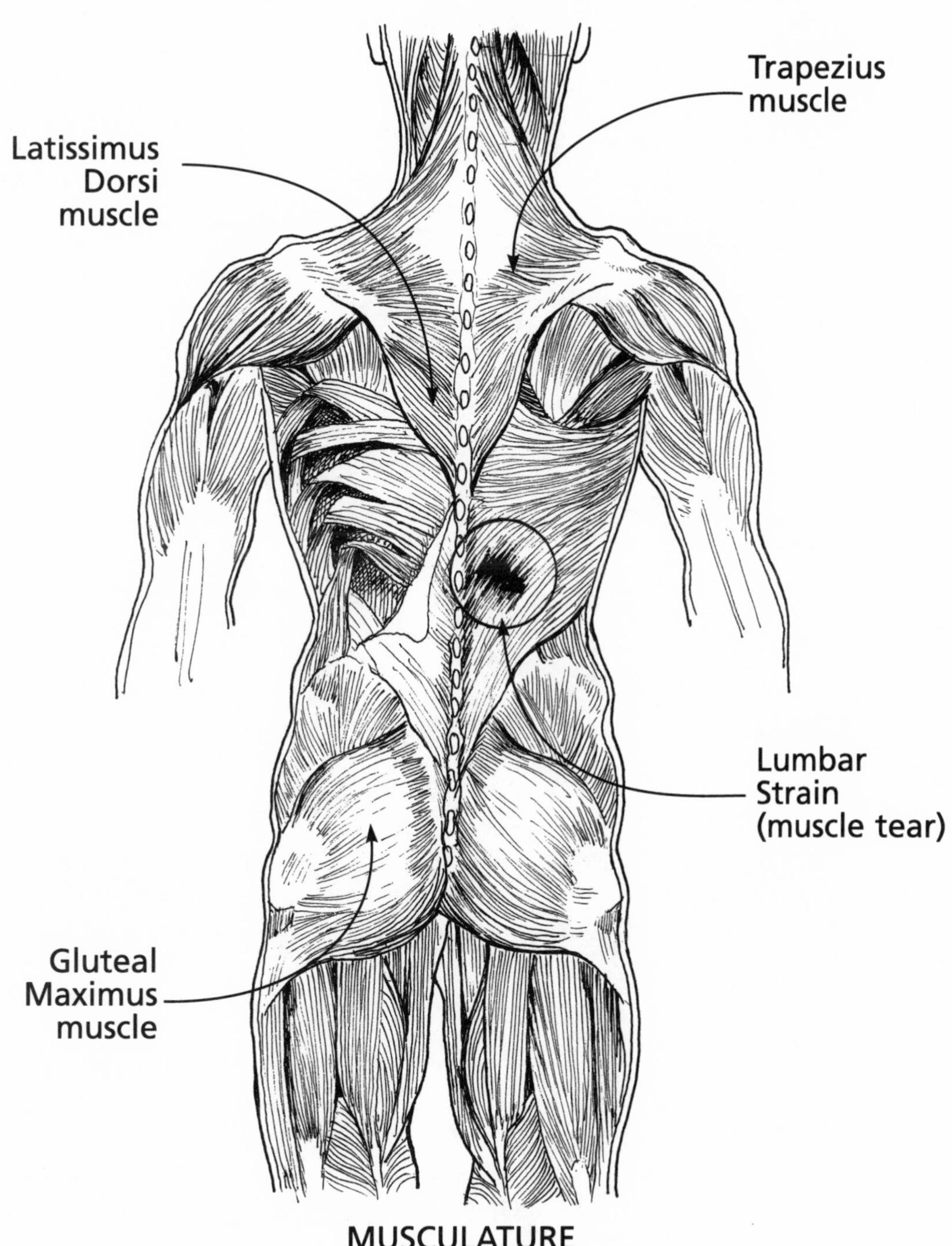

MUSCULATURE
(rear view)

Causes of Back Pain

Some Medical-Speak for Why Your Back Hurts

❍ MECHANICAL PROBLEMS

Back Strain

Overused muscles or ligaments which result in aches or spasms. Pain is usually located in the low back, buttocks or back of the thigh. Back strain can be caused by a specific motion or activity, single or repeated, or can be the result of poor posture. There are no diagnostic tests for back strain, but the area will be sore, pain will increase with activity and there will be an increase in muscle tension. It's estimated that 90% of all back pain is mechanical in origin, and that 60-70% of back pain episodes are the result of strain. Most back strain is treated conservatively, at least initially, with bedrest, mild pain relievers and traditional modalities.

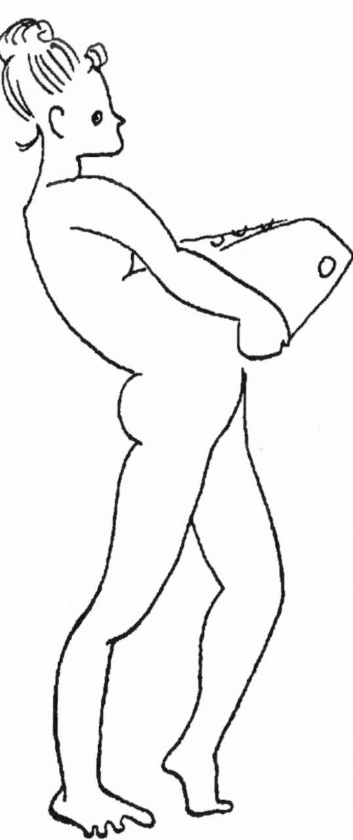

Herniated (or slipped) Discs

Discs are the rubbery, gel-filled cushions between the vertebrae. The gelatinous substance is held together by a fibrous covering called the annulus fibrosis, which is 90 layers thick. (In terms of structure, think of a jelly doughnut.) If this covering begins to weaken and thin out from damage cr injury, often from combined twisting and lifting of heavy objects, the gelatinous filling can begin to protrude toward the spinal canal. If some of the fibers rupture, rather than just weaken and thin, the filling can move further and extrude (herniate) into the spinal canal. This can cause pressure to be placed on the nerves of the spinal canal causing sharp, shooting or burning pain anywhere from the low back to the lower leg. Sciatica, pain from the large nerve that begins in the back and extends down the back of the leg, may occur years after a

§ *Stand tall, look ahead. If you forgot what good posture is, try standing with your back and heels against the wall. Check your shoulders and head – are they against the wall too? Try placing your hand at the small of your back (against the wall) and pushing on your hand with your lower back. Practice walking with this book on your head.*

herniation. It's worth noting that herniated discs can be present with no pain, depending on the relative size and location of the extrusion. Also, the discs shrink with age which makes herniated discs much more common in people aged 20-40, though this shrinkage creates a higher likelihood of degenerative problems.

Whiplash

A cervical spine injury, occuring when the head whips violently forward and then back, as it does in rear-end collisions. Ligament, muscle, nerve and soft tissue damage are most likely to occur. Pain is experienced most frequently at the base of the skull, and often behind the eyes, down the arms and/or in the shoulders or between the shoulder blades. Often the symptoms won't show up for 12-24 hours after the injury. Physicians will often use x-rays to determine the extent of the damage, and then prescribe non-steroidals like ibuprofen for pain and swelling, a neck brace and physical therapy. Neck braces may be helpful at first by limiting movement and thereby decreasing pain. But they may cause symptoms of their own. As you raise your shoulders during daily activity, the brace can can cause trapezius muscle spasm and/or irritate the base of the skull. Dependence on the brace can also weaken the neck muscles. Whether you wear a brace or not, chances are you will feel better within a few months. However, many whiplash victims state that 8-9 months later, the pain recurs. Degenerative changes in the cervical spine and minor neck pain are fairly common long term effects of whiplash.

❍ DEGENERATIVE STRUCTURAL CHANGES

Spinal Stenosis

A shrinking of the spinal canal. As the spinal canal shrinks, the nerves and the spinal cord become irritated and swell, which causes further irritation. This is often difficult to treat, and surgery is sometimes required to increase the size of the canal. Symptoms of spinal stenosis can closely mimic symptoms of angina (decreased circulation caused by shrinking blood vessels), including pain in the buttock, thigh or leg while walking. There is at least one telling difference between symptoms of angina and symptoms of spinal stenosis. While angina patients will experience pain while walking uphill or upstairs because of the physical exertion involved, spinal stenosis sufferers *will not* experience pain while walking uphill or upstairs. Spinal stenosis sufferers will, however, experience pain walking downhill or downstairs.

Bone Spurs (Osteophytes)

Irregular overgrowths of bone that grow on the spine to protect shrinking discs. These changes are a major cause of stiffness and backache in older people.

❍ ARTHRITIC AND RHEUMATIC CONDITIONS

Spondylitis (Osteoarthritis or Degenerative Arthritis)

A very common degenerative disease of the joints which involves chemical alterations in the cartilage, spinal stenosis (see above) and the development of osteophytes (see above). Studies have shown osteoarthritis to be present in nearly all individuals over the age of 75, though not all experience pain as a result. Common symptoms include low back and leg pain, often described as shooting, aching or pins and needles, and pain on walking or standing, usually relieved by rest. Osteoarthritis cannot be cured, but symptoms can be controlled with proper care.

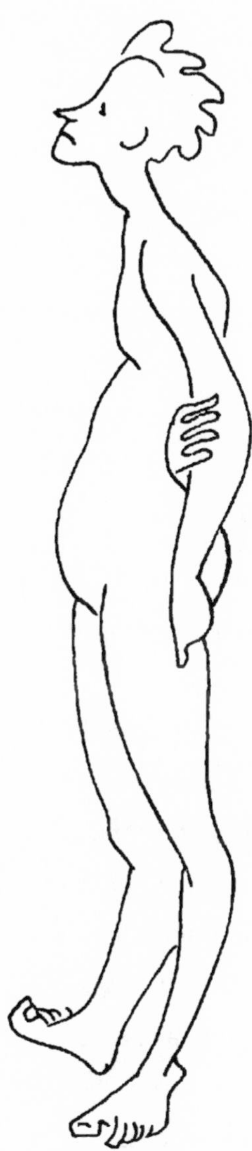

§ *Get help moving furniture – better yet, have others do it and you play director.*

Rheumatoid Arthritis

An inflammatory disease which causes pain, swelling, heat, and destruction of joints. If affects women approximately three times as often as men. It is significantly less common than osteoarthritis as a cause of back pain but more serious. It usually starts in the peripheral joints, like the fingers, but may spread to others causing visible deformity of the joints. By the time low back pain occurs, the disease has usually been present for a long time and the diagnosis is usually known. Inflammation and pain can be reduced with medications and, while the damage is largely irreparable, it can be kept under control.

Gouty Arthritis (Gout)

A condition more common to men than women. Uric acid, one of the primary components of urine, is not adequately excreted by the body. The acid accumulates in the joints causing pain.

Ankylosing Spondylitis

An inflammatory joint disease of the spine which is genetically related and about as common as rheumatoid arthritis (which is to say, only about 1-2% of the white population). The disease occurs in men approximately three times as often as women, and usually appears between the ages of 15 and 40. Morning stiffness and decreased motion are common symptoms. Back pain tends to begin in the low back, for months, but progresses to involve other parts of the spine and eventually creates a rigid spine and a posture in which there is no lumbar lordosis. (Lumbar lordosis is the normal sway in the lower back. The rigidness of the spine is what leads the condition to be referred to as poker spine or bamboo spine.) The disease is treated medically with exercises to maintain range of motion and flexibility, as well as pain reducing medications, though more intensive therapies are often employed as the disease progresses.

§ *Carry only what you need for the day. Use backpacks with the straps on both shoulders. Women should try not using a purse at all, or at least a very small one with only a comb, lipstick, license, and check-book. Now is the time to minimalize.*

Reiter's Syndrome

The most common arthritic condition in young men. Reiter's Syndrome is initiated by an infection, often gastrointestinal or venereal, in a person who is genetically predisposed to the condition. The disease is readily recognizable, as it is associated with a triad of symptoms: urethritis (inflammation of the end of the urinary tract), arthritis in the legs and back, and conjunctivitis (inflammation of the outside lining of the eye). The disease is not curable and its course is somewhat unpredictable. In 30-40% of those who have the disease, Reiter's syndrome lasts for 3 months to one year. In the rest, it develops a pattern of relapse and remission or continuing disease.

Polymyalgia Rheumatica (muscular rheumatism)

Rheumatism is the name applied to conditions that cause pain around the joints but that do not involve the joints themselves, in other words, non-arthritic pain around the joints. Rheumatism involves the muscles, tendons and ligaments. Polymyalgia Rheumatica is an aching pain usually with stiffness, most often in the upper shoulder girdle and neck area, but sometimes also affecting the low back, buttocks, and thighs. It occurs in older people, women four times more often than men, and can sometimes create inflammation of the blood vessels in the cranial area which can result in blindness.

Medical doctors usually treat this condition with steroids which reduce inflammation and control pain.

Fibrositis

A common cause of low back pain occuring, it is said, in compulsive, perfectionist people. It is associated with interference with sleep, morning stiffness, fatigue and tenderness, especially over the sacrum and shoulder area. Some studies have suggested that Fibrositis may be caused by disturbances of sleep which prevent normal restorative functions from occuring. Fibrositis cannot be detected by laboratory tests. It is believed to be an affliction of the connective tissue and muscles, but there is no proof.

§ *Make sure that any time you need to reach above your shoulders to get something, you're standing on a stepstool.*

Facet Joints

Recent research has suggested that irritation of the facet joints may be the predominant cause of low back pain. Injury to facet joints, the joints between the vertebrae which allow for spinal flexibility, causes inflammation, damages and thins the cartilage, and leads to new irregular bone formation (osteophytes) in the area. The joints may also become loose and may dislocate as they degenerate. Rotational stress (lifting and twisting), compression and muscular contractions, particularly of the multifidus (rotator muscle of the lumbar spine), may result in injury to these joints. Frequently, the same injury also affects the disc, forming a complex of damage. The complexity of the damage is probably the main reason for the uncertainty around the role facet joints actually play in causing back pain. It's difficult to detect what happens first.

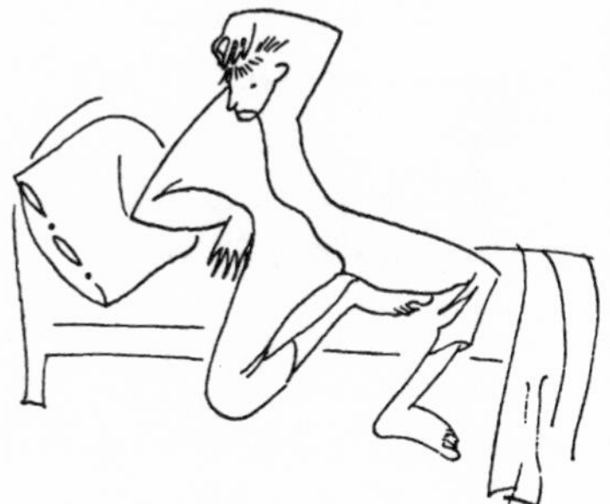

❍ MECHANICAL DEFECTS

Spondylolysis / Spondylolisthesis

These terms describe a structural condition of the vertebrae. Spondylolysis is a weakness or break in the lamina, the supporting base of the spinous processes, which may be genetic, structural or environmental. This occurs in approximately 5% of the population. Spondylolisthesis is the slippage or displacement of one vertebra on the other as a result of the weakness. These conditions often appear between ages 5 and 7 but will often cause no noticeable problems until much later in life. It is not clear whether or not these conditions

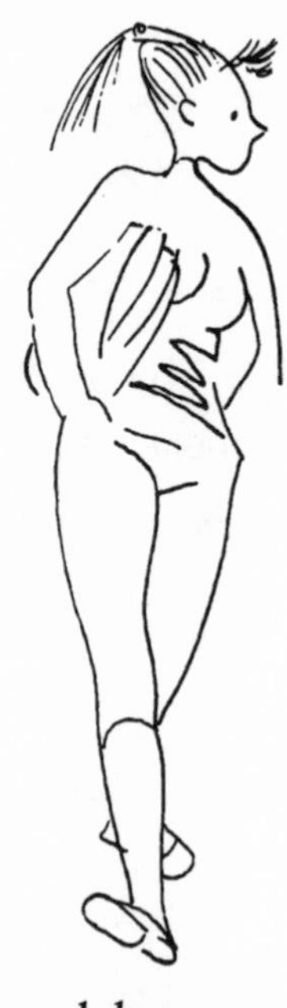

"As your abdomen expands, your abdominals become less effective at holding your spine erect. Your center of gravity changes and you may compensate by leaning back. This can stir up back troubles. Be sure not to stand with locked knees (it exagerates a sway back), and keep your pelvis tucked in a pelvic tilt. . . . Postpregnancy, learn how to lift, handle and carry your baby using your legs and arms rather than your back. It takes time to get muscles toned and ligaments shortened, so take it easy for the first six weeks after delivery."

– *Glamour*

actually cause back pain. There are usually other associated changes – disc, facet joints, *etc.* – and some people with the defect experience no discomfort at all. Those who do will often experience pain as an ache in the low back, thigh or lower leg beginning with a specific movement (like twisting and lifting) or injury.

Leg Length Discrepancy

If one leg is shorter than the other by greater than half an inch, the pelvis will be tilted. To compensate, the spine tends to shift toward the shorter leg. If allowed to go unresolved by the use of a shoe lift, this imbalance can result in painful structural changes to other parts of the body: ligaments, muscles, tendons, discs, knees, legs and pelvis.

❍ CONDITIONS COMMON TO WOMEN

Osteoporosis

Decrease in bone density, common in post-menopausal women, which leaves the bones vulnerable to fracture. According to recent studies, 33% of women over age 65 have vertebral fractures because of osteoporosis. Hip fractures are also extremely common, effecting approximately one-third of all elderly women and one-sixth of all elderly men at some point in their lives. Risk factors for osteoporosis include aging, menopause (especially early onset), smoking, high alcohol consumption and family history. White and Asian women are most vulnerable to the disease because, generally speaking, they have the lightest skeletons (lowest bone density at maturity). Osteoporosis is caused primarily by a lack of calcium in the bone matter. However, bone formation and bone loss are "ballistic"; that is, the more calcium you put in early in life, the longer it takes to run out. Thus, preventive medicine for osteoporosis includes increasing your calcium intake before aging and hormonal changes set in. Exercise for men, and for women both before and after menopause, can help increase and then maintain bone mass. Other risk factors for osteoporosis include Chronic Obstructive Pulmonary Disease (COPD), leanness, and possibly high protein intake which may negatively effect calcium absorption.

Pregnancy – During and After

Pregnancy produces a decided shift in a woman's center of gravity, increasing weight in front and causing extra pressure on the discs of the lower back. Pregnancy also causes the release of hormones which relax the ligaments, ideal for delivery but not for working, walking, and everything else you do in the meantime. Post partum women are also extremely vulnerable to back problems due to weakened abdominal muscles which do not adequately support the lower back. Delivery as well can cause back pain for some women if the movement of the baby creates pressure on the nerves of the back. Exercise to maintain muscle tone in the abdomen and using a pelvic tilt position can help, as well as rest and good general body mechanics (especially after you give birth and spend your time lifting and carrying the new baby) can help make the natural effects of pregnancy less burdensome on your back.

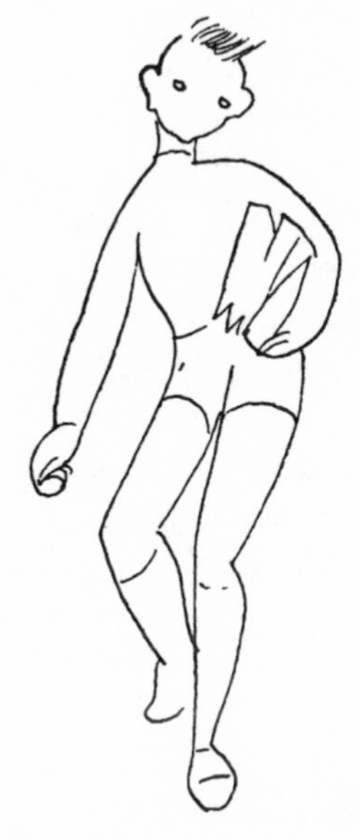

❍ SPINAL CURVATURE

Scoliosis

A lateral (sideways) curvature of the lumbar spine, greater than 10%. Scoliosis is far more common in women than in men, and if the curve is less than 40%, it is usually asymptomatic and requires no treatment. If greater than 40%, a brace can be used on younger people to prevent progress of the curvature. In adults, a brace is unlikely to be effective. If the damage is severe, and the pain is unremitting, more radical corrective measures may be recommended. Adults with scoliosis may experience aching pain or fatigue in the lumbar section of their back.

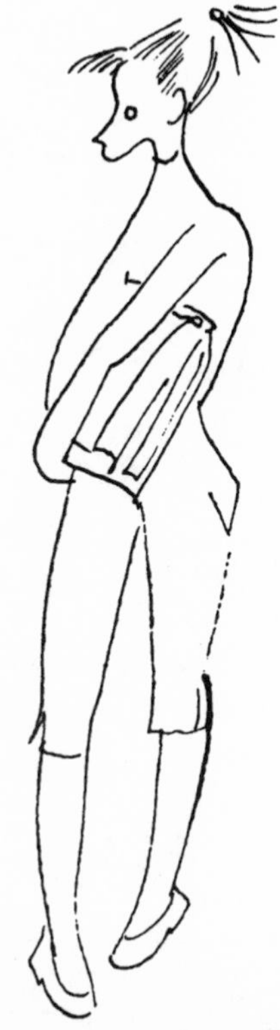

Kyphosis

An excessive forward curve of the spine at the shoulder blades, usually angular with wedging of the vertebrae. This is less common than scoliosis but more serious, and most likely to become serious in young girls. It can be caused in older people by osteoporosis. It was once a common result of spinal tuberculosis but now it is more commonly caused by Osteochondritis (see below). Victor Hugo's Hunchback of Notre Dame is probably the most famous case of Kyphosis.

"Back pain is serious, even if you've only had it once. Most first-time back pain sufferers don't give their backs much thought once the pain has subsided. They jump right back into life, doing nothing to keep their backs healthy. . . Back pain is something that must be taken seriously. It is a sign of weakness in the bones, discs or muscles of the spine and back."
— Arthur White, *Shape*

Lordosis

An exaggeration of the normal lumbar curve of the back (swayback). Only extreme lordosis is associated with back problems.

Vertebral Osteochondritis (Scheuerman's Disease, Juvenile Kyphosis)

A condition which primarily affects teenagers. Changes at the junction of the vertebrae and discs of the thoracic spine create increased curvature (kyphosis), with pain in the thoracic area. If left untreated, kyphosis may increase, pain may persist, and compression of the spinal cord may occur. Treatment of Vertebral Osteochondritis usually involves the use of brace until the patient has stopped growing to prevent deformity from occuring.

❍ INFECTIONS

Vertebral Osteomyelitis

An infection of the vertebral bone caused by any number of organisms, often the result of an infection in another part of the body, like a respiratory or urinary tract infection. Osteomyelitis usually attacks the lumbar spine or sacrum and is often experienced as a sharp ache in that area, accompanied by fever and general illness or malaise. The course of the illness varies greatly depending on the organism involved but, once diagnosed, it can usually be treated with antibiotics and bedrest.

Herpes Zoster (Shingles)

Herpes Zoster may cause pain on one or the other side of the back for several days, along with fever and sometimes gastrointestinal symptoms, before a characteristic blistering rash appears to reveal the diagnosis. Herpes Zoster is a late occuring complication of Chicken Pox. The pain from this condition is a neuralgia and is often experienced as burning, sharp, deep, or tingling. While this condition often resolves itself with no further complications, older people may experience persistent pain. Treatment mainly involves pain control, though, depending on the age and health of a patient, doctors may prescribe other medications to prevent complications.

❍ OTHER CAUSES OF BACK PAIN

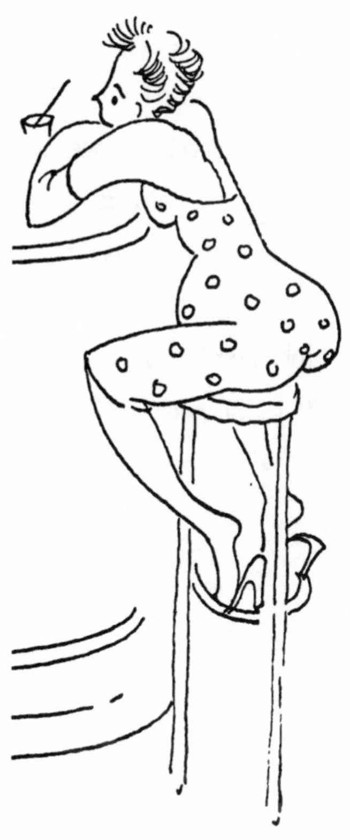

Referred Pain

This is an important consideration in thinking about back pain. Referred pain in the back, that is, pain generated by a problem in another area but experienced in the back, can be caused by a wide variety of disorders. Some disorders, like abdominal aneurysms, for example, will sometimes generate back pain and are dangerous if not diagnosed. Kidney problems are often associated with back pain, usually causing pain in the flank. An early misdiagnosis of ovarian cancer as a back problem is not uncommon. It's important to be attentive to other symptoms in addition to back pain, as well as the location of the pain, in order to obtain a proper diagnosis.

Psychiatric

Some back pain can be caused by or exacerbated by what physicians categorize as psychiatric conditions. Chronic back pain can produce a set of symptoms diagnosable in medical terms as clinical depression. The loss of appetite, change in sleep patterns, anxiety and inactivity associated with chronic back pain can contribute to progressive depression which can then contribute to the pain itself. In other fairly rare cases, psychiatric illness, like psychoses or schizophrenia, can manifest back pain as one of its symptoms. In these instances, a medical doctor will usually perform extensive testing to rule out any organic cause of pain and then refer a patient to psychiatric care. Anxiety and hysterical conversion (the unconscious transformation of an emotional problem into a physical dysfunction) would also officially fall into the category of psychiatric ailments, though these clearly take place with greater and lesser degrees of severity. Not everyone who experiences back pain in response to anxiety or stress is mentally ill. Rather, studies of these problems provide clinical support to the general wisdom that stress and other mental and emotional conditions have profound impacts on the ways in which people experience their bodies.

§ *Do plan time to exercise, do yoga, tai chi, or meditate sometime in each day. Exercise and meditation are wonderful stress reducers.*

Tumors

Though among the most unusual causes of back pain, tumors are also among the most serious. Tumors often reveal themselves in persistent back pain that increases in reclining positions. Different kinds

§ *A duster with a long telescoping pole should help those with spider webs in the corners of the room. Or a clean towel wrapped a broom, if it's long enough.*

of tumors, however, both benign and malignant, will progress in different ways and, therefore, manifest different symptoms. With some types of tumors, for example, aspirin will provide temporary pain relief while with others, aspirin will have no effect. Standard laboratory tests are not particularly helpful in diagnosing tumors of the back, but many tests, including CT Scans and MRIs, are extremely effective in locating lesions (see Diagnostic Tests). Early diagnosis can prove particularly important in the successful treatment of tumors.

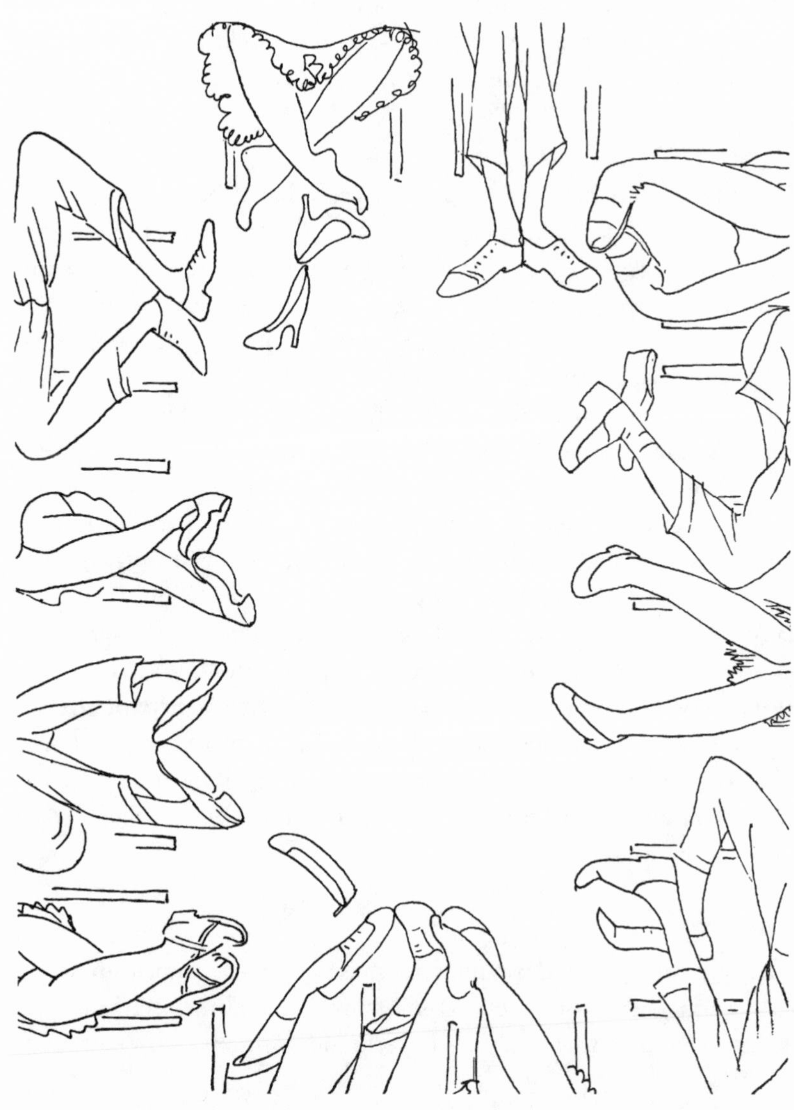

HEALTH PRACTITIONERS

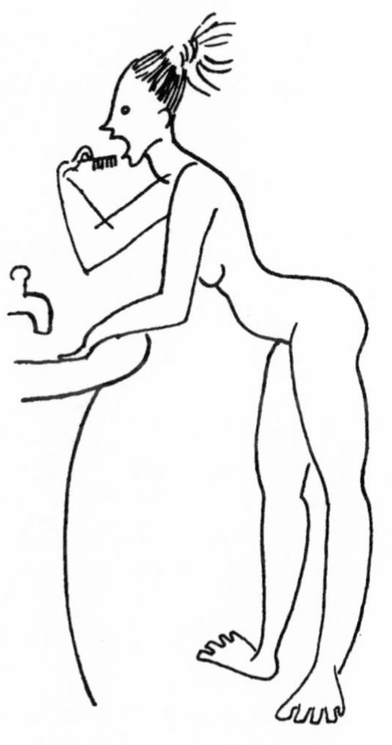

Acupuncturist

These are licensed health care professionals. They use the ancient art of Chinese acupuncture. Thin needles are used to locate and treat pain, following a system of body meridians. Make sure the acupuncturist is well qualified. (Ask about their training – they should have completed a licensed training course. In Korea, doctors have vigorous medical training, and internship and then specialize in acupuncture). Different states have different laws concerning acupuncture.

Chiropractors

These are not MD's. They are licensed health care professionals. Their specialty is spinal manipulation. They cannot prescribe drugs nor work in most hospitals. As with any practitioner, it is best to let a chiropractor know what level of pain you're in, so he or she can use as gentle a touch as you require. Sometimes spinal manipulation can involve vigorous treatments. More Americans go to see chiropractors for low back pain than any other type of health care worker, much to the ire of the medical profession. They are also the best at short term relief of pain, according to one study.

General Practioner (G.P.)

A medical doctor that practices general medicine. If you have a good family doctor whom you've been seeing for years, and he or she can recommend and work with other specialists or physical therapists, this could be the best situation. G.P.'s are in the best position to know all about you. Unfortunately, most G.P.'s alone can do little more than request x-rays, and prescribe medication, which may or may not address the causes of your back problems. They can, however, rule out serious illness and give needed referrals to physical therapists, back schools, or specialists.

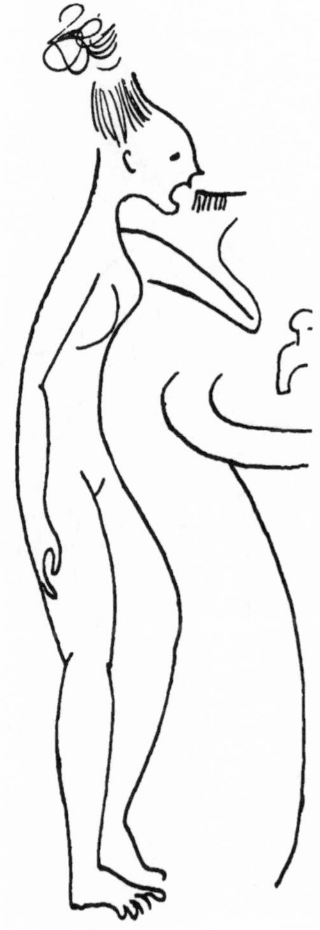

Herbalists

Could refer patients to chiropractors or osteopaths for manipulation. They recommend herbal remedies for well being and to aid in healing. Chinese herbal medicine is often used in conjunction with acupuncture.

Kinesiologist

chiropractor who has studied both chiropractics and kinesiology (the study of mechanics and anatomy in relation to body movement). Often these specialists will be able to show you how to move, stand and sit in an optimal position. They (like herbalists and chiropractors) are more interested in a holistic approach to your health, including diet, work, exercise and relationships.

Neurosurgeon

Medical doctors specializing in surgery of the nervous structures: brain, spinal cord, *etc.* Neurosurgeons don't treat general back problems except surgically. They are unlikely to be experienced in long term back rehabilitation. Their track record is the highest for prescribing drugs, not just painkillers, but also anti-depressants.

Osteopaths

Doctor of Osteopathy. These are MD's with extra years of specialty in skeletal manipulation. Osteopaths can prescribe drugs and perform surgery. Osteopathy is a system of medical practice based on the theory that disease is due to the loss of structural integrity and through manipulations of the spine, health can be restored.

Orthopedic surgeons

These are MD's with a specialty in surgery for disorders of bones, muscles and joints. If a laminectomy or fusion is necessary you will be referred to one of these doctors. Some orthodpedic surgeons seem uninterested in cases not requiring surgery, or if there is nothing showing up on the x-ray. Since large city surgeons can command large salaries, they realize that time is money. Don't settle for less than attentive, caring, listening orthopedist, willing to treat soft tissue problems as well. Your time in pain and the state of your back take precedent to the surgeon's salary. You have a right to expect that you will get the best medical care.

§ *Hire help. Help is cheaper than hospitals*

Physiatrists

MD's that specialize in rehabilitation medicine. They are more likely to prescribe an exercise program, and referral to a physical therapist.

Physical Therapists

These are not doctors. They have a college degree in physical therapy and they are professional health care workers. Their job is to follow out the recommended treatment program suggested by a medical doctor. Often this time is scheduled for so many minutes of ice, heat, traction or ultrasound. Physical therapists that work closely with back schools or pain clinics often teach work and daily living rehabilitation programs designed to help clients to change the everyday aspects of their lives that are hard on the back.

Sports Medicine Specialist

Sports medicine is not a certified medical specialty. Any medical doctor, orthopedic surgeon or chiropractor can call themselves a specialist in sports medicine. It is best to ask them, before you make an appointment, what experience they have in treating athletes or injuries in your sport. How many years have they been treating sports injuries? What percentage of their practice is really sports related? Do they belong to any professional groups like the American College of Sports Medicine or the American Osteopathic Academy of Sports?

cathy® **by Cathy Guisewite**

"MANY PEOPLE TENSE THEIR BACK MUSCLES INSTEAD OF EXPRESSING ANXIETIES AND FEARS, WHICH WEAKENS THE MUSCLES AND MAKES THE BACK VULNERABLE TO INJURIES."... THIS IS YOU, IRVING!
THAT ISN'T ME, CATHY.
BACK PAIN
"BACK PAIN IS CAUSED NOT SO MUCH FROM LIFTING ONE THING WRONG AS IT IS FROM A LIFETIME OF DENYING FEELINGS BY CLENCHING THE BACK."....THIS IS YOU!
THAT IS NOT ME!
NOT ME! NOT ME! NOT ME!
BAM BAM BAM
...OUCH.
"EMOTIONAL PAIN THAT GOES UN-ACKNOWLEDGED WILL SURFACE SOMEWHERE AS PHYSICAL PAIN..."

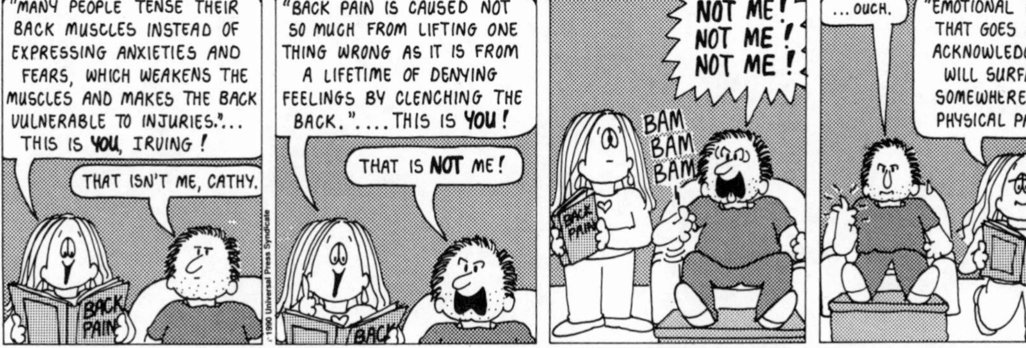

WHAT WORKS

In a survey of 492 back pain sufferers which sought to determine the effectiveness of back pain treatments, Arthur C. Klein and Dava Sobel came up with some enlightening results. Their book, Backache Relief, ***will likely be of great interest, especially to those who have already been through the mill on their backs. We highly recommend Klein and Sobel's unique and extremely important commentary on the available methods of back care. Their approach, which encourages back pain sufferers to explore their options and take control of their health care, accords with the philosophy that motivated this book. We find their book thorough in its analysis, and rich with useful, detailed information.***

According to the survey respondents, practitioners most likely to deliver moderate or dramatic long-term help were yoga instructors, physical fitness instructors, dance instructors and physiatrists. 82-96%* of those who tried the first three of these methods (51 total respondents) experienced predominantly dramatic long-term success, though only yoga managed to leave no one feeling worse. Physiatrists performed extremely well for the fairly small number who visited them. 86% received long-term help, though 53% described the help as moderate rather than dramatic. Klein and Sobel note, however, that unlike yoga or dance, a physiatrist's treatment can be utilized by those with severe or incapacitating pain.

"Since women lack upper arm strength, they carry weight with their neck, shoulders and upper back. That can translate into back stiffness and pain. The big offenders: heavy shoulder bags, overloaded plastic grocery bags and overstuffed briefcases."
— *Glamour*

Chiropractors and orthopedists were clearly the most sought after practitioners, visited by 422 and 429 of the 492 respondents respectively. One-third of those who visited chiropractors found the

*All percentages presented here are approximate

treatment ineffective, and slightly fewer received some temporary relief. Nearly a third received moderate or dramatic long-term help. 61% found orthopedists ineffective, however, and, though only 7% felt worse after receiving orthopedic care, only 23% received any long term benefits. Of all the practitioners, neurologists fared worst, providing 76% of their back pain patients with ineffective treatment, and leaving a full 16% feeling worse than before they came.

Of the drugs used by back pain sufferers, aspirin provided the most frequent temporary help (78%), followed by tranquilizers and muscle relaxants (36% each). Tranquilizers and prescription anti-inflammatories were most likely to make patients feel worse. The largest proportion of drug therapy was deemed ineffective, with virtually no long term benefits.

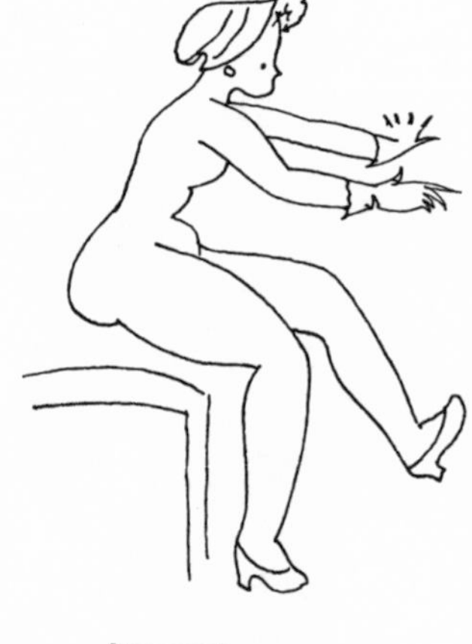

Of standard therapies – manipulation, heat, traction, massage, braces, *etc.* – traditional back exercises provided the greatest number of people (77% of the 278 respondents) with moderate or dramatic long-term help. Manipulation, though tried by 333 of the 492 respondents, provided long term help for only 12%. Traction proved by far the least helpful to survey respondents. While 22% received temporary relief, 52% found it ineffective and 24% felt worse.

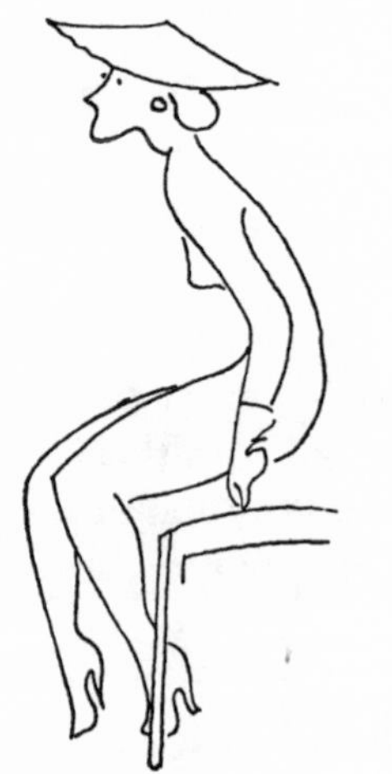

The more controversial treatments had fewer takers overall. Of the 65 patients who had surgery, 25% found it dramatically helpful, 25% found it moderately helpful, 28% got some short term relief, 8% found it ineffective and 14% found it worsened their condition. Foot orthotics (shoe inserts, *etc.*), gravity inversion and biofeedback all provided a high percentage of users with long-term benefits, though the actual numbers remain fairly small.

It is worth noting here that all of the treatments and practitioners listed in *Backache Relief* helped somebody in some way. Even treatments that made some people feel worse provided others with dramatic long-term benefits. Statistics can thus provide only so much information, and they can't substitute for experience. But that information can be wisely used, and if these statistics reveal anything important, it is that treatment which involves active participation – yoga, exercise, dance – is most likely to yield dramatic long-term results for sufferers of mild to moderate back pain.

For more extensive statistical information, along with analysis and excerpts from respondent interviews, see *Backache Relief* (Times Books (Random House), 1985). It's a source not to be missed.

RELIEF AT HAND

Back Pain and Manual Medicine

By Sarah Key

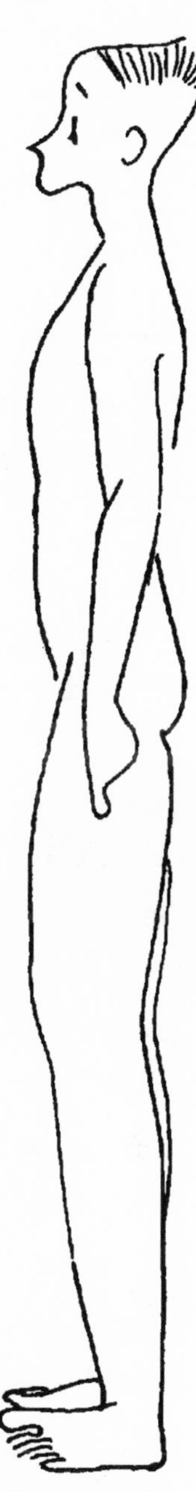

The stupefying grandeur of the human spine almost defies description – let alone explanation. It is the most marvelous working instrument, incomprehensibly more delicate, sophisticated and finely tuned than any Stradivarius violin, and yet it doesn't cost a million dollars and all of us have one.

It's probably because the spine works so well that we take it all for granted – until it starts causing trouble, usually pain. And then everything becomes shrouded in a blur of mystique. No explanations, sort of mute concern. You put up with the problem and we'll do the worrying about it. Odds-on we all inherit this sort of bother anyway – being human and upright and all that. Everybody seems to shrug their shoulders. Those who suffer wander off without purpose and without hope; the only companion to their pain, a sheaf of x-rays and a bottle of pills and some indistinct date in the future to see the doctor again. In the meantime, they have been subjected to an endless routine of diagnostic procedures with scant even perfunctory attention to therapeutics. All tests and no cure. And so there they all go with their crooked spines, wandering in a wilderness, waiting for some providential guidance towards the light.

I can't quite explain this hubris within the profession. Except that it is a very daunting spectacle to witness a fellow human cast down by a serious back problem. What practitioner will ever forget his or her first patient crippled in this way; as if that wretched back had taken on a will of its own, the patient a weakened and terrified victim in its path? It's easy to do nothing; not to interfere and aggravate things and to suggest that 'time' and 'rest' take their natural course. That's the non-interventionist's approach. And then, of course, there is the massive intervention of spinal surgery; when that beautifully subtle and succinct mechanism is tampered with by knives and chisels and other fearsome tools.

§ *Bring reading material up to your eyes. Don't drop your head. A slantboard (purchased at a hospital supply store or, better yet, a store specializing in back products) can be used at home for doing bills, reading, and writing letters. If your job entails scheduling work, it can be a godsend. The podium, with its slanted surface and standing height is perfect. If you use a sloped drafting table, make sure you have a chair high enough.*

My own area of therapeutic interest is the No Man's Land between these two extremes. That half-way place where the magic sensibilities of human touch meld with the awesomely delicate machinery of Nature's own most awesome and delicate machine. Of course, I always flout danger using words like 'magic.' Within the realms of conventional Western Medicine, I know the risks I run when I talk about healing, not therapy, and when I eschew the help of x-rays, or CAT scans, or MRI's and the like. It is just that I have the dual resources of human feel and human touch at hand and I find, as the years fold by, that this tells me more of what I have to know – what is wrong and what has to be done – than the shining impersonal armory of chromium-winking lights which deliver rays and magnetism and other sorts of science fiction 'tests.'

Increasingly in the way I work, I know that I hover at the edge of professional acceptability and I cannot say that I am completely inured to the eyebrows askance of my own professional kith and kin. But as I delve away and tinker, probing and focused with thumbs nudging at the exquisite nuts and bolts of this fantastic willowy column, I know that I have deliberately taken myself back out of the unlearning process which coerced me – like the educated adult who has lost the innate wisdom of childhood – to forget my instincts in search of knowledge. Of course, I am aware that I challenge conventional thinking as I shed the strictures and the cramping edicts of scientific wisdom and abandon myself to the calm and the quiet where real healing begins. I do not see myself as a faith healer or a conduit of any other persuasion. It is just that I see, as time goes by, that in the laying on of hands, the simpler one keeps it, the better. The less flamboyant the academic posturing, the better.

I attend to the human spine by feeling around in it with the hands. I use the skills of a manual therapist or manipulative therapist and for me, 'feel' is everything. Such a forgotten notion that; human hands on, using the sensibilities I was born with. In fact, I am often amused by that; in this age of space travel and biogenetics and lasers and any other of the unintelligible 'things modern,' I do exactly the same today in tending to a painful spine that I would have done as a caveman. . . or cavewoman perhaps.

§ *Sit down to put on shoes and socks or stockings.*

Human thumbs are perfectly designed to probe about in the nooks and crannies of a spine. Rather like a well-tuned musical instrument, a normal healthy spine will resonate or 'go with the flow' of normal probing pressures. If there are any linkage problems with the spine, they are immediately apparent because they can be felt. Not only do the problem joints not slide away from the investigating thumbs, they remain querulously rigid, defiant to approaching pressure, and this pressure also hurts. Thumbs can also pick up swelling, thickening and local muscle spasm deep in and around the joints of the spine. Marvelous that, don't you think? And quite apart from that, from the patient's point of view, it also feels so comforting to have the problem found, actually touched. Just in the same way that an anxious patient will absent-mindedly rub the painful part of her spine as she goes about explaining the problem, the dysfunctional part of the spine is actually helped by this local pressure. This local accurate movement is just exactly the sort of pressure needed to initiate the cure.

Simply speaking, this is what I do. Through feel, I look for anomalies in the freedom of all the spinal vertebrae. If any of them are loathe to go in one, or several, directions, this will constitute a function fault and will be a source of pain. This is the fundamental tenet in the ethos of Manual or Manipulative Medicine.

If you came to see me, I would examine you by lying you prone over a pillow so that your spine was relaxed and floppy and, with graduated pressures, I would cruise around, looking for faults in the segmental mobility. To watch it, it would look as if I were running my fingers up and down a keyboard. I would ease and tug at each vertebra in turn, from every different direction, reverent in my fingertip respect. I might find, for example, that a vertebra was free to glide forwards on the vertebra below but that it had completely lost its ability to swivel from left to right, or vice versa. Or, it may swivel well enough but when I applied the forward gliding pressure on its neighbor below, it moved forwards unevenly, sluing around as it went, by being tethered at one side at the back by a malfunctioning facet joint. All technical stuff and also very subtle to feel.

But the important point is that over time, simple function faults such as these play havoc in the ability of the spine to defray strain and act out its role smoothly. Sooner or later there will be pain.

§ *Get a broom and dustpan with long handles. A godsend!*

The most common variety of back pain is the result of the simple vertebral impaction just described. Like one stiff link in a bicycle chain, it is indeed surprising how much pain this sort of thing can bring. It is usually a centralized low-grade ache and on local pressure, the problem vertebra itself often feels like a bruised bone.

In the low back, other more serious conditions can develop in the course of a degenerative sequence. What starts off as a simple jamming may eventually effect the intervertebral disc, for example. The disc starts to suffer when it is deprived of the pumping-bellows effect created by the squeeze and wheeze of its two flanking vertebrae. Since a disc does not have the benefit of its own blood supply, it is intimately dependent upon flourishing, grandiose movement of the spinal segments to suck in and expel nutrients. The freer the vertebral mobility, the greater the alternating pressures within the disc and the more efficient the pump.

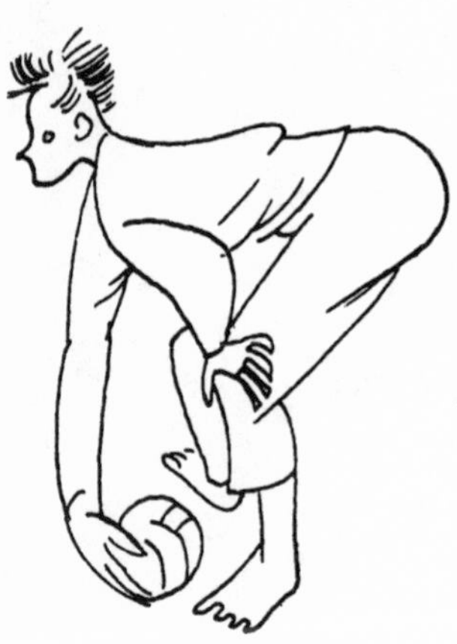

As a spinal segment loses mobility, the pump imbibition of the disc loses gusto. The disc loses nourishment; it shrivels and drops in height and loses some of its inherent ability to act as a shock absorbing roundel between its two vertebrae. Its walls weaken and eventually bulges or herniated discs appear – the whole downhill story. In some parts of the disc wall, the bulge itself can be painful and you can also get pain as these bulges impinge on the sensitive spinal nerve lying close by. The pain in this instance is sciatica or pain in the leg, but you can also get more of the simple back ache, the first pain described above, simply from the increased vertebral impaction as the disc loses height.

The third source of pain is another development in the sequence: degeneration of the facet joints. The apophyseal or facet joints can suffer increased wear and tear as the water content of the disc decreases. In their normal state, the two opposing surfaces of these joints (two of which sit sentry-like at the back of each disc) nudge into each other and form a bony lock. This neighborly restraint prevents the movement of any one vertebra going too far. But if the interceding disc deflates like a juicy pillow losing its bounce, the two opposing surfaces of the facet joint over-ride on each other as the segments ram closer together. The superincumbent vertebra sinks down on to the one below and sets up a long term grinding of the facet joints – in fancy language known as lumbar spondylosis. This causes a nasty local pain in the back, or on the side of the joint affected. There may also be referred pain over the buttock and perhaps down the upper thigh.

And finally, the picture of advanced dysfunction: the acute locking back. As the jammed segment and collapsing interceding disc deteriorate further, the spine alternates between being as stiff as a board and giving way at the slightest provocation. Shrinkage of the intervening disc leaves a latent instability of the facet joint which guards that disc. A facade of brittle stiffness overlies a latent sloppiness of the link. In the machinery of the spine there lurks a weak link, ready to fail whenever the spine is put to the test. Although you may go on for years before anything comes to light, at some point some chance awkward movement may bring you down. A sneeze say, and you are caught as if cast in bronze, by an agonizing sear of pain through the back. The latent slackness of the soft tissues was unable to bind the spine securely together. For the most part you are not bothered by it. You get around with your back stiff and you never bend to lift. Then some unavoidable movement and you find that the fine intersegmental control is not there. You are incapacitated; on the floor and having to crawl to your bed and the telephone. Apart from the acute pain from the wrenched facet joint, you may have enough swelling of this joint also to impinge on the close-lying sciatic nerve and cause sciatica.

§ When you get into a car, make sure there is nothing in your hands. Heavy packages, bags, etc. should be put in the trunk. When you get into the car, turn around facing away from the car and sit down in the seat. Swing your legs into the car only after you are sitting down.

So you can see from the summary of four of the most common forms of back trouble, that the fundamental problem lies in the sluggish mobility of a spinal segment. The good news is that not only can this be identified by feel through human hands, but those very same hands can hold the cure.

By thoughtful manual pressure, it is possible to free the impacted segment, or the one impacted freedom of a segment. Rather like coaxing a rusty link in a bicycle chain back to noiseless free-hinging function, it is possible to coax a stiff vertebral link back to full painless freedom. With an action akin to prizing a champagne cork out of its bottle, exerting a pushing and releasing pressure, over several treatment sessions, it is possible to restore full segmental mobility. This is known as manual mobilization of the spine.

§ *Keep the most often used and heaviest items at waist level.*

About the Author:

Sarah Key has been treating the human spine for over two decades. She practices out of her physiotherapy clinics in Sydney, Australia and London, England, where she treats patients from all over the world. Her book, *Back In Action,* with a foreword by one of her best known patients, His Royal Highness, the Prince of Wales, is now in its third edition. To be published by BBC Books this year, in conjunction with a BBC series of the same name, is *Body in Action,* a do-it-yourself action kit on maintenance of your own jointed skeleton. The book and series discuss proper function, problems and preventive care of all the joints in the body. Sarah Key is also the author of *Freddie: Diary of a Cot Death* [Heinemann (UK/Aust.) 1991]. She lives in Sydney with her husband, Russell Keddie, and her three children Jemima, 11, Harry, 9, and Scarlett, 3.

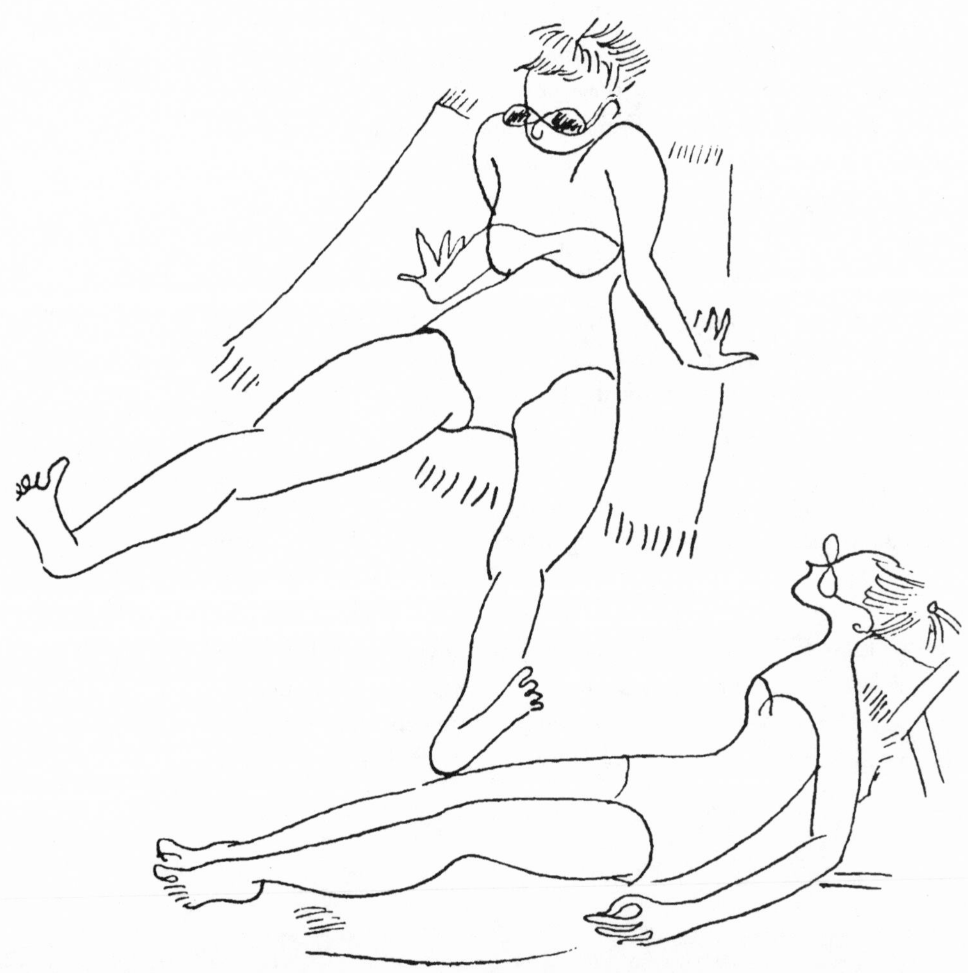

THE MEDICAL DOCTOR'S VISIT

When you visit a doctor for back pain, providing precise information and specific answers to questions will help you to obtain a quick and accurate diagnosis. It will probably help if you think about the answers ahead of time.

It is very important to characterize the pain in several ways. Precisely where is the pain? To where does it travel (radiate)? Describe the pain. Is it an ache, a sharp pain, a burning sensation, or some other feeling? When does it occur (day, night, periodically, unpredictably)? What brings it on (an activity, a movement, certain positions)? What relieves it (rest, standing still, sitting, lying down, urinating, aspirin, Tylenol, another medication, heat, or whatever)?

The history of the back pain is important. How long have you had the pain? When was the first time? Describe the circumstances. Were you engaged in a specific activity or movement? Were you ill in some other way? Have you had recurrent episodes? Under what circumstances? Have you had tests, x-rays or treatment? When? Where? What were the results?

"The best way around back pain is to work toward proper posture. Proper posture is a learned, athletic skill, like any athletic skill, it involves muscular support and awareness."
— McCloy and Taggart, *Women's Sports and Fitness*

Your general medical and social history may be related to your current complaints. What illnesses, accidents or operations have you had? Do you take medication? (Don't forget home remedies, vitamins, birth control pills, *etc.*) Have you taken medicine in the past? Were you hospitalized? When? Where? What for? (Old records may contain useful information.) Do you smoke? Drink? What is your occupation? What are your leisure activities?

What is your family history? Has anyone in your family had back problems? What kind? In addition, don't hesitate to add any information which you feel may be related.

Though this seems like a lot of information, a medical doctor will need all of this in order to rule out any life threatening causes of back pain, and other serious illness. He or she will probably order a blood test if arthritis is suspected, and will ultimately rely on standard tests for mobility, reflexes, strength of muscles, flexibility, a straight leg raise to check the sciatic nerve, and touch to check for areas of pain.

§ *Make sure you have or can install a shower. Getting in and down and up and out of a bathtub on a regular basis is a pain in the back and can cause even more pain in neck injury situations.*

If the pain seems to be caused by strain or overworked muscles, bed rest might be recommended from 3 days to 2 weeks. Physical therapy is often prescribed in addition to or instead of bed rest, depending on the severity of the problem. Find out if there might be a back school you can attend (see Back Schools). Most back schools require a doctor's prescription because back schools incorporate physical therapy with re-education on proper movement, and other modalitites.

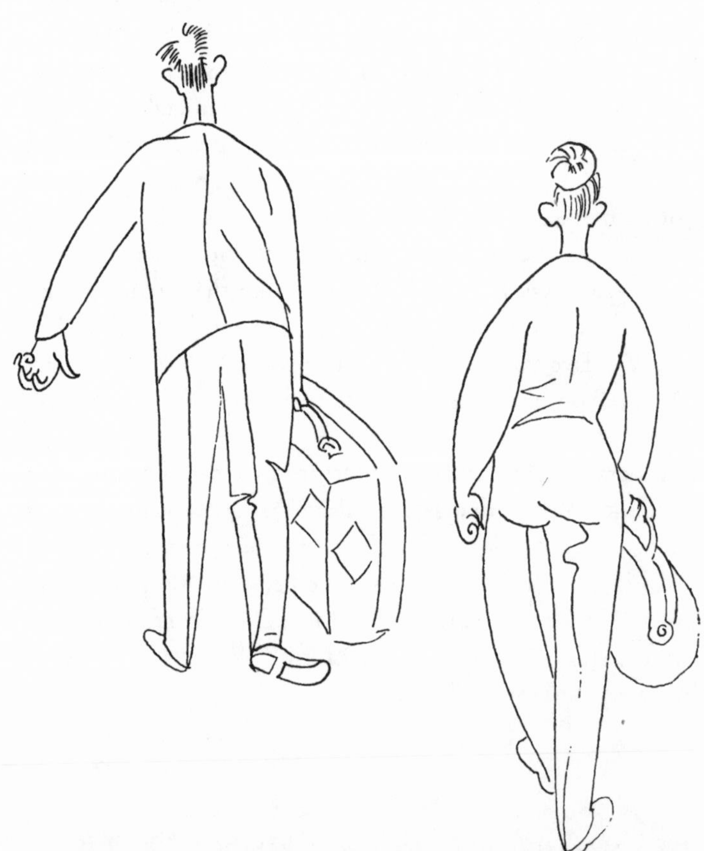

CHIROPRACTICS

In 1988, the American Medical Association withdrew its condemnation of Chiropractic as a cult, in order to comply with federal rules pertaining to fair trade. Cooperation between medical and chiropractic professionals is increasing, though the AMA as a professional organization is still resistant. In a report released by the RAND Corporation in July 1991, however, a panel of leading physicians, osteopaths and chiropractors found chiropractic care was helpful in treating low back pain in those people who had recently experienced back pain but were otherwise generally healthy.

HERMAN®

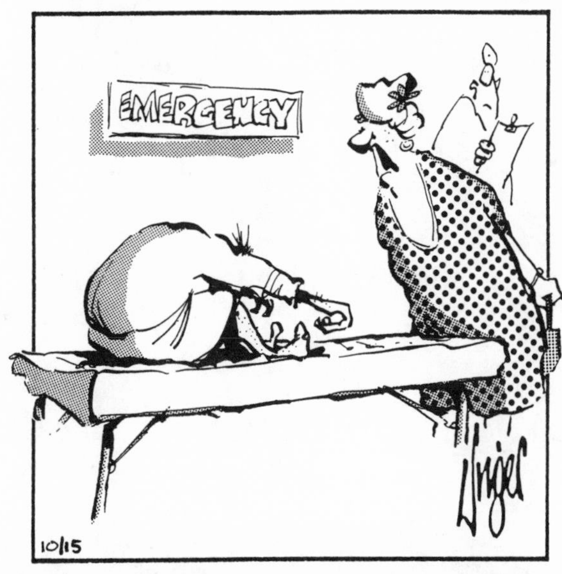

"I *told* you not to use a rowing machine."

CHIROPRACTIC AND YOUR BACK

William C. Meeker, D.C., M.P.H.
Thomas B. Milus, D.C., D.A.B.C.O.

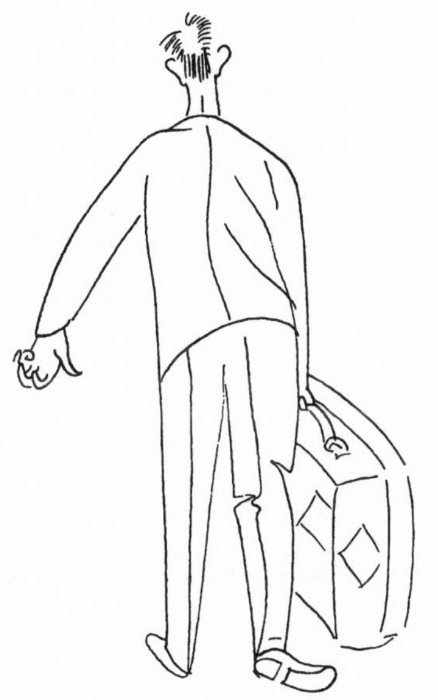

THE PROFESSION OF CHIROPRACTIC

With 45,000 members, the profession of chiropractic comprises the second largest group of health professionals after medical physicians. Today, after a history of 100 years, Doctors of Chiropractic (D.C.) provide care for about ten percent of the population annually in the United States. Many patients choose chiropractors for their reputation in treating back problems. In fact, chiropractic physicians treat thirty percent of all patients with back pain in the United States. The prestigious RAND Corporation has estimated that two-thirds of all health care visits for back pain are to chiropractors.

The modern Doctor of Chiropractic is a highly trained professional. Chiropractors must receive at least six years of undergraduate and post-graduate training, very similar to a medical school curriculum, at colleges accredited by an agency officially recognized by the United States Department of Education. Doctors of Chiropractic are licensed in all 50 states only after passing rigorous state-controlled examinations. Many chiropractors also receive additional specialty training and certification in such topics as orthopedics, neurology, nutrition, radiology, and sports medicine.

THE CHIROPRACTIC APPROACH

Chiropractic care is traditionally conservative, drugless and non-surgical. It is a profession that believes in the inherent healing powers of the body and emphasizes overall body wellness in maintaining a healthy back. Chiropractors treat with a variety of mostly "hands-on"

§ *Get store workers to help you out to your car with large packages or groceries. Also ask them to bag your groceries lightly. Even if you have help getting it into your car, you need to be able to get them out. It is excruciating to carry packages that are too heavy and it takes all day to take items out of the bags and carry them into the house one by one.*

adjustive, manipulative and physiological procedures. Physiotherapy modalities such as ultrasound, muscle stimulation and traction are also applied as each patient's case warrants. The Doctor of Chiropractic usually couples the program of treatments with a plan for home care including such things as stretching, strengthening, exercise, dietary recommendations, and healthy lifestyle enhancement. Doctors of Chiropractic recognize that many factors contribute to health.

When you go to a chiropractor, you can expect to be in a setting similar to a medical office. You can expect to receive a consultation with the doctor concerning the reason for your visit to the office. He or she will want to know about your past medical history. Your doctor will perform a general examination if indicated, and a detailed examination of your area of complaint. A spinal examination is performed to assess the movement and other characteristics of your joints. The chiropractor also assesses, for example, the skin, muscles, and ligaments. These have the potential for contributing to your back pain problem. Abnormalities in these tissues might provide clues to the underlying cause for your pain. In many cases, x-rays are ordered to assist in an accurate diagnosis and the design of an effective treatment plan. In more difficult cases your doctor may order other sophisticated tests, such as magnetic resonance imaging (MRI) or computed tomography (CT scan).

The causes of back pain are numerous. Your Doctor of Chiropractic knows how to diagnose and manage sprains and strains, sacroiliac joint dysfunctions, intervertebral disc conditions, sciatica, myofascial (muscle) pain, facet syndromes, postural abnormalities and those conditions resulting from industrial and other accidents.

After making a diagnosis, the chiropractor decides how to handle treatment of the problem. You should expect to receive a clear explanation of the diagnosis and the course of care your chiropractor feels will best help you. Should you need a referral to a chiropractic or medical specialist, your chiropractor should explain that process and help you make the arrangements.

Unlike the not so distant past, there is a growing level of cooperation and respect between the medical and chiropractic communities when it comes to treating back pain. Patients with complicated or very severe spinal conditions are often best managed by such a professional "multidisciplinary team approach."

❍ THE SPINAL ADJUSTMENT: THE MOST IMPORTANT CHIROPRACTIC TREATMENT

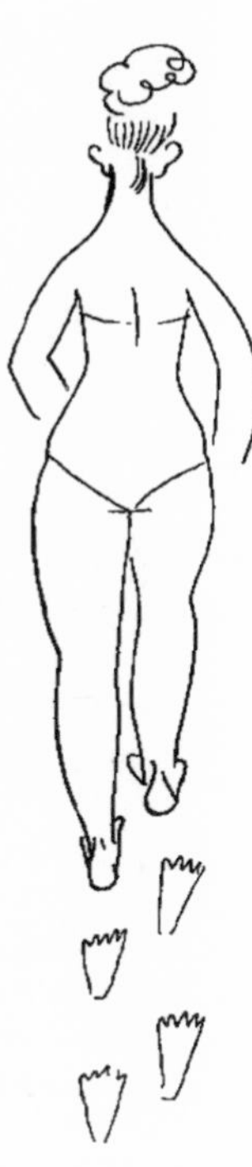

Adjustments and manipulations of the spine and other joints have existed as a remedy throughout history. In the United States, it has been the chiropractic profession that has kept alive the art and tradition of this effective procedure. Today, while a number of health professionals claim to use spinal adjustments and manipulations, Doctors of Chiropractic remain the most trained, the most skilled, and the most experienced in this area of knowledge.

Chiropractors use the word "subluxation" to describe the problem that exists when a joint does not function properly. The assessment of abnormal joint function during the physical examination includes the movement of the joint, the presence of pain, muscle tightness, swelling, redness, visible structural abnormalities, *etc.* The x-ray is often used to assist the evaluation of these joint problems. In addition to surveying the x-rays for signs of serious pathology (disease), the chiropractor checks for signs of joint degeneration which may indicate abnormal joint movement.

The Doctor of Chiropractic usually performs a manual "adjustment" to remove the subluxation, in an attempt to restore normal joint function. The adjustment has traditionally been described as a high-velocity, low-amplitude thrust. In plain language, this means the chiropractor skillfully and quickly applies a small, highly controlled force to the body.

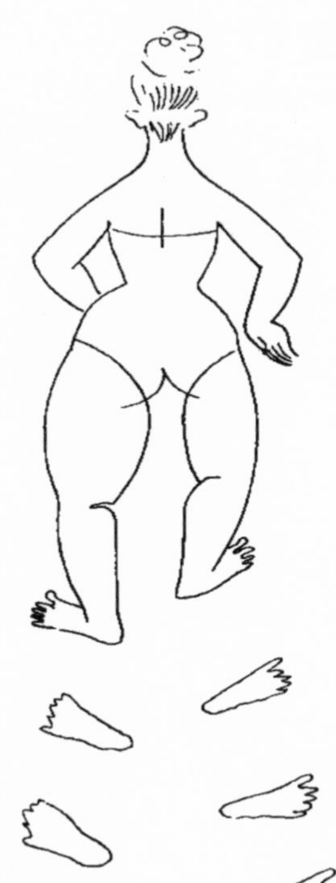

The most well-known method of performing an adjustment to the low back has the patient lying on his or her side. The doctor stands in front of the patient and stabilizes the patient's shoulder. The doctor reaches behind the patient and applies the adjustive procedure to a specific joint in the back. Another approach has the patient lying face-down while the doctor applies the adjustment to the joint. This maneuver may be assisted mechanically by a specially designed piece of equipment located directly under the patient. A third method of treatment employs small wedges placed under the patient's pelvis while lying face-down or face-up depending on the intended effect. A fourth major category of treatments employs manual pressure upon and stretching of muscles and other soft tissues.

In cases of intervertebral disc complaints, the famous "slipped disc," a specialized table may be employed which offers a stretching force to assist in eliminating the problem. Chiropractors do not

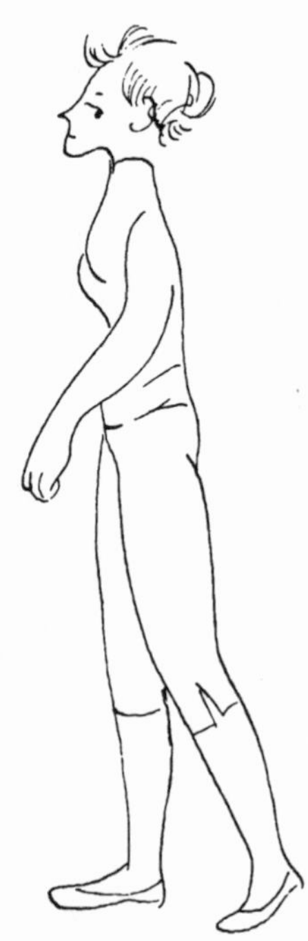

believe that the entire disc actually "slips" although a part of the disc may actually become displaced.

Your recovery is based upon the type of problem, its severity, and its chronicity. Long-standing back pain generally takes longer to realize improvement. Similarly, just as a sprained ankle takes longer to heal than a sore muscle from working in the yard, certain conditions take longer to treat than others. There are, however, some guidelines you may use. If your condition is going to respond to chiropractic care you should see results within a one to two month period. Often Doctors of Chiropractic will treat a condition three times per week for two to four weeks and then evaluate your progress. It is important that you follow your chiropractor's recommendations for exercise and other home care instructions to achieve the best results.

WHAT DOES SCIENTIFIC RESEARCH TELL US?

In this age of consumer awareness, patients are rightfully asking their doctors to explain the scientific evidence justifying their methods. In this section, some of the recent research on chiropractic will be described. Interested readers can find more detail in the references at the end of the chapter.

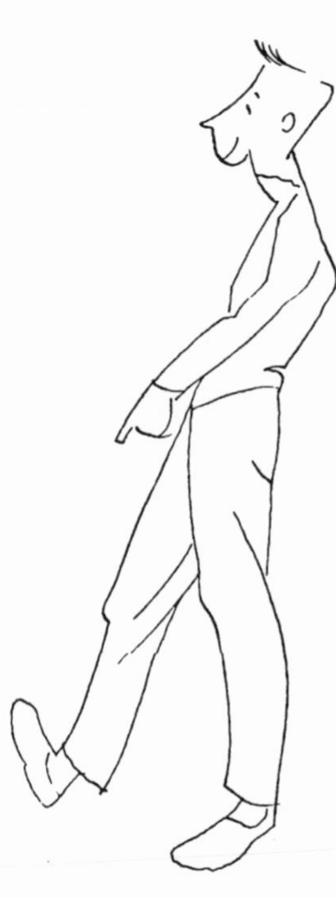

The RAND Corporation, a prestigious health care "think tank," recently published a report on the appropriateness of spinal manipulation for low back pain. In that effort the researchers identified over twenty controlled clinical trials and over fifty additional scientific studies. The consensus of a nine-member expert panel consisting of medical, chiropractic and osteopathic experts concluded that spinal manipulation was an appropriate treatment for common forms of low back pain. What is most surprising to many, including many medical physicians, is that spinal manipulation may be the most thoroughly studied treatment for back pain that exists.

Recently, the British Medical Journal published a study comparing outpatient chiropractic care to care delivered in the standard British health system. Chiropractic patients demonstrated a greater reduction in pain and disability than their medically treated counterparts. For the patients that were studied, this held true even after two years.

In another interesting study, researchers found that medical and chiropractic physicians held distinctly different attitudes about their ability to manage back pain. Essentially, Doctors of Chiropractic had greater levels of confidence and felt more well-trained in this area than the medical physicians who were studied. In a related study, patients were surveyed for their attitudes with respect to chiropractic and medical treatment for their back pain. The group of chiropractic patients reported satisfaction levels three times greater than the medically treated patients.

§ *Install handrails on the wall to use as you enter your tub.*

Notwithstanding the explosion of spinal research in the past decade, the problem of back pain is still widespread. A large number of scientific issues still need to be resolved with additional research. Many studies are now in progress. Chiropractic does not have all the answers, but the scientific community is now ready to admit that chiropractic has a great deal to offer the individual with low back pain.

❍ REIMBURSEMENT FOR CHIROPRACTIC CARE

All fifty states authorize chiropractic services under their Workers' Compensation programs. The majority of states also require inclusion of chiropractic services under major commercial health and accident policies written in those states. Most plans treat chiropractic claims as they would any other medical claim. At the federal level, chiropractic services are covered to varying degrees under Medicare and Medicaid programs. Most private and self-insured employee insurance programs also enjoy coverage of chiropractic services. Patients should check their particular policies to ascertain the extent chiropractic services may be covered for them.

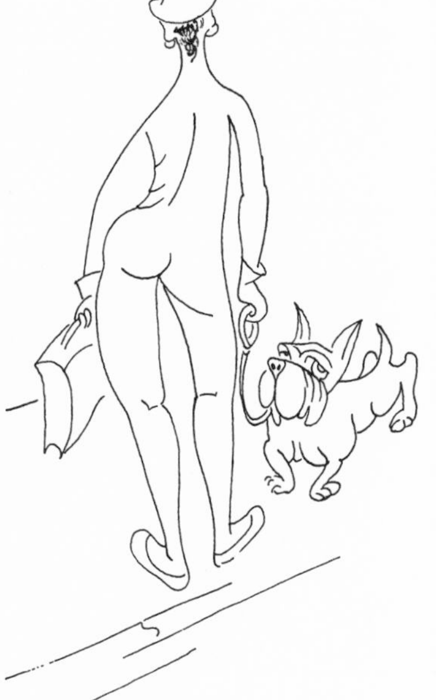

❍ CHOOSING A DOCTOR OF CHIROPRACTIC

As with the choice of any doctor, your decision should be based upon a level of investigation into who is qualified in your area. Referral by a trusted friend or family member is a method often used. Selecting a doctor from the telephone book or any advertisement may be satisfactory but is not recommended. A personal referral is more likely to provide a satisfactory doctor. Keep in mind that selecting a doctor is a process which may take time. If you do not feel comfortable with a particular Doctor of Chiropractic, seek additional referrals in your community.

REFERENCES AND SOURCES FOR ADDITIONAL INFORMATION

American Back Society. 2647 E. 14th St., Oakland, CA 94601

American Chiropractic Association. 1701 Clarendon Blvd., Arlington, VA 22209

Cherkin, D, McCormack, F: Patient Evaluation of Low Back Pain Care from Family Physicians and Chiropractors. *Western Journal of Medicine* 150: 351-355, 1989.

Consortium for Chiropractic Research. 1095 Dunford Way, Sunnyvale CA 94087

Foundation for Chiropracitc Education and Research. 1701 Clarendon Blvd., Arlington, VA 22209

Haldeman, S. (ed): *Principles and Practice of Chiropractic* (2nd Edition). Norwalk, CT: Appleton and Lange, 1992.

Meade, T, *et al*: "Low Back Pain of Mechanical Origin: Randomised Comparison of Chiropractic and Outpatient Treatment." *British Medical Journal* 300: 1431-1437, 1990.

Kirkaldy-Willis, W., Cassidy, J: "Spinal Manipulation in the Treatment of Low-Back Pain." Canadian Family Physician 31:535-540, 1985.

Shekelle, P., *et al*: *The Appropriateness of Spinal Manipulation for Low-Back Pain, Project Overview and Literature Review*. Santa Monica, CA: RAND Publication R-4025/1-CCR/FCER, 1991.

Shekelle, P., *et al*: *The Appropriateness of Spinal Manipulation for Low-Back Pain, Indications and Ratings by a Multidisciplinary Expert Panel*. Santa Monica, CA: RAND Publication R-4025/2-CCR/FCER, 1991.

"For every 29-cent stamp you stick on a letter, three cents goes to pay for back ailments suffered by postal employees. Only the common cold leads to more missed workdays than backaches do."
– Joseph Alper, *Washington Post Health*

About the Authors:

Dr. William C. Meeker is the Dean of Research at Palmer College of Chiropractic-West in Sunnyvale, California, and the President of the Consortium for Chiropractic Research. He is on the Board of Directors of the American Back Society and holds several distinguished editorial positions. He is the Principal Investigator of a number of ongoing spinal research projects.

Dr. Thomas B. Milus is an Associate Professor of Clinical Sciences at Palmer College of Chiropractic-West and a Clinical Professor in the outpatient clinic at the college. He is board certified by the American Board of Chiropractic Orthopedists (D.A.B.C.O.) and by the American Academy of Pain Management (D.A.A.P.M.).

Conservative Treatment

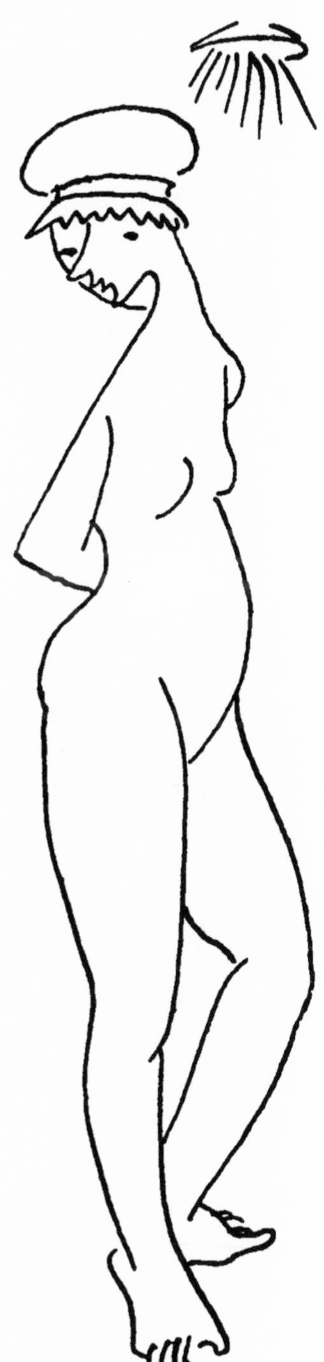

❍ TRADITIONAL MODALITIES

These are things done to you on your body surface, usually by a physical therapist, that are expected to have a deep effect. Heat, cold, traction, ultrasound, massage, and hydrotherapy all fall under this category in a typical hospital physical therapy department.

These may allow you time to relax, and thus feel better, but they probably will not cure you. Ice has its place in the first 48 hours after a muscle strain, and heat can provide wonderful, soothing relief from a nagging backache, but they don't solve the problem. It is ultimately up to you to take care of yourself by attending to the causes of your back problem.

❍ TENS-TRANSCUTANEOUS ELECTRICAL NERVE STIMULATION

TENS is a battery operated pack (like a Walkman) that you attach to your waist. There are wires that attach, not to headphones, but to patches that are placed on either side of your spine. These patches contain electrodes. When you feel pain you can turn up the frequency to "jam" the pain receptors to your brain.

A recent study published in *New England Journal of Medicine* found no beneficial effect directly connected to TENS machines. This form of treatment, however, is widely used by well-reputed treatment centers and is accepted by major insurance companies and medicare.

❍ CONSERVATIVE TREATMENT ALTERNATIVES

ALTERNATIVE BODYWORK METHODS: Alexander Technique, Mensendieck, Trager, Rolfing, Massage

Alexander Technique

Named after F. Matthias Alexander, a Shakespearean recitalist born in 1869, who discovered a way to improve his hoarse voice. He realized that the way he held his head in relation to his neck and back affected his voice. Rather than finding discs or muscles to blame for our pain, Alexander Technique instructors teach us how to recognize patterns of tension created in the ways we currently sit, stand and move. According to this method, if we are in pain, we are likely doing something to interfere with the proper balance of energy in our bodies, and performing movements in ways that use energy inefficiently. Alexander Technique has been described as psycho-physical therapy. You learn to feel how you are holding your body, and how to develop more control over your movements. (For more information, contact North American Society of Teachers of the Alexander Technique. See Resources.)

"If you have a bad back, it's essential to work on general spine flexibility; this means knee-to-chest stretching exercises, pelvic tilts and abdominal-strength maneuvers such as modified sit-ups."
– Ruthan Brodsky, *New Choices*

Mensendieck Exercises

Dr. Bess Mensendieck, born in 1861, was an opera singer, sculptor and doctor. Her experiences in these fields led her to establish a method of personalized therapy where individuals develop a body-sense of good posture and muscular awareness using exercises that emphasize stronger muscle tone and correct muscular coordination, but also accomplish active relaxation. Among her pupils were Greta Garbo, Ingrid Bergman, Frederic March, Mrs. Fred Astaire, Mrs. Irving Berlin, and Mrs. Gary Cooper. Her method of kinesiology therapy (the only one dealing with the mechanics of the joints) is still widely used in Scandinavian countries. Teachers are required to train in a two year specialized course of study and work one-on-one with the patient. (See Mensendieck and You)

Bodywork Therapy

The following are not so much forms of physical therapy in the traditional sense, but are more philosophies or healing arts.

Training programs usually require a certain number of hours before the person can become certified or be a practitioner. Each one has its followers. Some of the techniques are quite vigorous, some gentle. When in doubt, ask around to see what has worked for others. Certainly a calm, gentle, theraputic massage can leave you feeling relaxed and maybe even painfree. (For more information, contact the American Massage Therapy Association. See Resources.)

Trager Psychophysical Integration – the principles on which it is based were discovered by Milton Trager, MD, over 50 years ago. Manipulation of the body is used to re-educate the body as to what it feels like to feel alive, pain free, and be able to move more freely. It is a therapy that is done to you.

Acupressure and Shiatsu – both are done with finger pressure using a system of meridians (like acupuncture) to balance the flow of energy through the body. Shiatsu (a Japanese healing art) can also employ kneading with the elbows, or the fingers together.

Swedish massage – probably the most well known form of massage. Dating back to the 18th century to a Swedish man named Peter Ling. It is used to stimulate the blood through slapping, kneading, deep tissue massage and pounding.

Esalen massage – developed at Esalen Institute in California, it is a calmer, more flowing form of massage. The idea is to have the person being worked on, feel relaxed, calm and have a good experience.

Rolfing – named after Ida Rolf, who started her "deep conective tissue therapy" in the the 1940's. It is a vigorous, pounding form of therapy. If your pain is severe, this may not be for you.

Reflexology/Zone Therapy – massage for the feet which uses a system of correspondence between points on the feet and the rest of the body. You can try this yourself by getting a reflexology card at your local health food or herb store, and massaging the soles of your feet with your finger tips on the points recommended for your ailment. (Better yet, have someone else give you a foot massage). Intuitive and Sensitive Massage-focuses more on the intuition and awareness level of the person giving the massage, and what they and you feel is needed. This can be a very therapeutic massage for working on muscles and soft tissue problems.

§ *Get outlet or power strips. Place them at waist level above your existing outlets in each room, so you don't have to bend over to plug in or take out electrical cords, (or crawl under desks, behind couches etc.). Over time you will appreciate the difference this can make in your life, especially for weekly chores like vacuuming which requires plugging the cord in and pulling it out in each room.*

ACUPUNCTURE

An ancient healing system which uses needles inserted at specified points on the body. Acupuncture can greatly relieve pain, by an involved process of body meridians and the theory of chi (or the flow

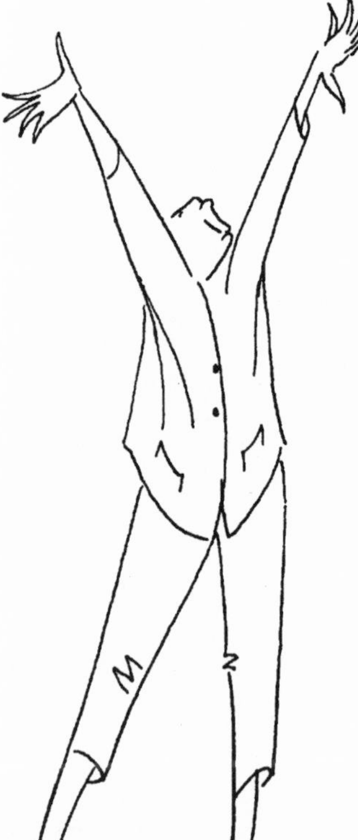

of energy in a body). Western medical studies have attributed the effects of acupuncture to the stimulation of endorphins, the body's natural painkillers (see section on Pain), but this is not conclusive. Frightening as the thought of a lot of needles in you at one time may be, they are very, very thin and it is a relatively painless procedure. Injection needles hurt because they have to be thick enough for liquid to flow through them. Acupuncture can't make your back situation worse, and it might be worth a few tries for low back pain and sciatica.

Make sure that the needles are sterilized or are disposable, to eliminate the possibility of the transmission of infectious diseases.

HYPNOSIS

A method of inducing a trance which makes a person more vulnerable to suggestion. Hypnosis has been used successfully in the treatment of pain, presumably by activating the body's own pain relief mechanisms (endorphins – see section on Pain). Usually done by doctors or psychologists once a diagnosis has been made.

RELAXATION TECHNIQUES

A variety of techniques designed to induce a deep state of relaxation in which respiration and heart rates decrease and muscles release tension. While not usually curative in themselves, these are often employed by physio-therapists, occupational therapists or incorporated into a Back School curricula to provide temporary relief from pain and enhance the effectiveness of other therapies. Relaxation techniques may be used in conjunction with a Bio-feedback machine. Outside of the clinic or hospital setting, relaxation techniques are used by meditators, yoga practioners, and atheletes to name a few, to help them obtain a relaxed state before continuing with their practices.

TAI CHI

A set of Chinese exercises aimed at improving endurance, flexibility and balance. The smooth, fluid motions of Tai Chi make the practice excellent for those who have been through back surgery or who are currently experiencing pain. Tai chi has been found to improve flexibility and stamina in the elderly.

§ *You might also want to install a handrail that slopes up toward your pillow on your bed. Especially if you have had back surgery, or are about to.*

DIAGNOSTIC TESTS

❍ X-RAY

An x-ray essentially shows only bone. It doesn't show discs, soft tissue and nerves. It cannot directly show a muscle spasm. Most spinal tumors do not show up on an x-ray. It will show fractures, bone spurs, scoliosis or a vertebrae that has slipped (spondylolisthesis) or a vertebrae with a defect (spondylolysis). It can also show when a change occurs in a normal segmentation of lumbar and sacral regions.

When you leave a doctor make sure that your x-rays go with you, or that your doctor is willing to send them to your next doctor.

The risk of x-rays is exposure to increased levels of radiation. Sex organs are very close to the low back and are more sensitive than any other part of the body to radiation.

Pregnant women should not have x-rays due to radiation exposure unless the benefits clearly outweigh the risks.

Pros

- ◇ *If a doctor thinks it could be one of the above problems, this is a relatively inexpensive test.*

Cons

- ◇ *If you suspect a disc or strain, it won't show up. Due to the radiation used in x-rays, cell damage may occur.*

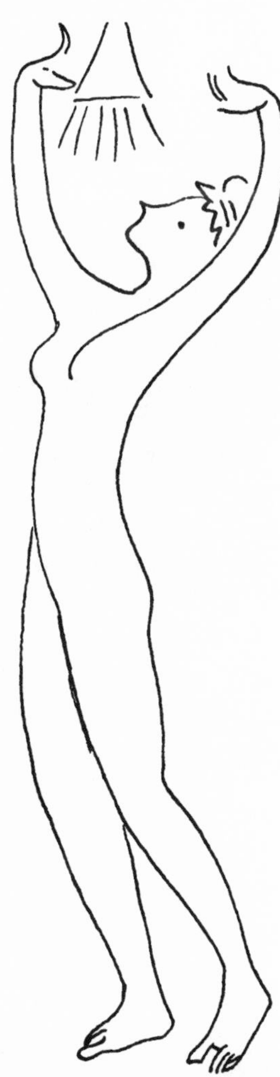

❍ EMG (electromyelography)

Tiny fine wires are inserted into muscles and nerves and then are electrically stimulated to test their level of function.

Pros

- *If a ruptured disc is suspected, an abnormal EMG may help confirm that diagnosis. Indication of nerve damage can be traced to nerve bundles coming off the spine and may indicate which disc is affected. It can show muscle and nerve damage. There is no exposure to radiation.*

Cons

- *There is often disagreement involving the interpretation of the readings. Pain level for the 1-2 hour procedure ranges from uncomfortable to excruciating even though the needles are very fine. There can also be some bruising.*

❍ CT scan or CAT scan (Computer Axial Tomography)

A computer generated three-dimensional image from a series of x-rays.

Pros

- *A CAT scan reveals a cross-section of the area. Herniated discs are visible. Spinal stenosis (narrowing of the central canal) can be seen. Tumors are visible as are degenerative bone diseases. Also visible is the spinal cord and spinal infections.*
- *Painless except for laying on your back on a hard cold surface. You go through a huge white arch. The test seems more foreboding than it is.*

"Prevention is probably the most effective strategy for reducing the tremendous costs and suffering associated with LBP [Low Back Pain]."
– John Frymoyer, MD

Cons

- *CAT scans are generally available only at major medical centers and are very costly. Sometimes CAT scans are not immediately available.*
- *Patient is exposed to radiation.*
- *May not differentiate herniated disc from postoperative scarring.*

❍ MRI (Magnetic Resonance Imaging)

This test is conducted without radiation. The patient lies within a large magnet which attracts electrical charges from your body. A computer collects these impulses and reconstructs an image of the area.

Pros

- ◇ *MRI's show soft tissue clearly (a herniated disc, disc degeneration, and ruptured discs), as well as bone, muscle and nerves (although bones are not as clearly defined as in other tests like x-rays). It can also show cartilage, ligaments, tendons, and blood vessels. This test is painless and is currently considered the "gold standard."*

Cons

- ◇ *The cavities in your teeth may hum uncomfortably.*
- ◇ *It cannot be used for patients with any sort of metal implant or pacemaker. The procedure requires that the patient lie still within a tube for up to an hour-not for the claustrophobic.*
- ◇ *Extremely costly. This test is more expensive than a CT scan. Many insurance companies are reluctant to pay for such an expensive test so check first.*

§ *Leave car mechanic work to the car mechanics. There is a Mechanic's Backsaver (see Back Designs in the Catalog Section) that might help with some tasks. Mechanics often complain of constant back pain from car work where bending, lifting, and twisting are a part of their lives. If this is your occupation, you need to do everything you can to reduce the torque and pain.*

❍ MYLEOGRAM

In this procedure the patient is placed on a table which tilts and a small quantity of spinal fluid is removed and replaced by an x-ray dye. The table is tilted to disperse the dye and x-rays are taken. Myleograms are used to diagnois the exact degree of disc herniation. Many doctors follow a myleogram with a CAT scan while the dye is still present in the spinal column to pinpoint the exact location, degree of the herniation and show its impingement on a spinal nerve. At this point in time, myleography is still widely used immediately before surgery where CT scans and MRI are not available to pinpoint the herniation.

Pros

- ◇ *Precision in pinpointing condition.*

Cons

- ◇ *With the advent of CT scans and MRI's, myleograms are not as frequently required as they once were. Myleograms can cause pain and complications in some patients, such as arachnoiditis which is an inflammation of connective tissue surrounding the spinal cord. Some patients experience headaches for some time. In general, myleograms should be performed only as a last resort. And not at all if you are unwilling to have surgery.*

- *(To lessen the chances of ill effects, drinking large amounts of fluids prior to the myleogram and having IV fluids before the procedure dilutes the dye as it enters the blood stream and speeds its departure via the urine.)*
- *Sitting up in bed for 8 hours after the procedure keeps the dye in the lower back and prevents it from traveling to your head where it can precipitate nausea and headaches.*

DISCOGRAM

This is an x-ray in which dye is inserted by a needle into the suspected disc(s) and monitored by a radiologist. In a normal disc the dye has no way to escape and shows up as a blob inside the disc. If the disc is herniated the dye will leak out.

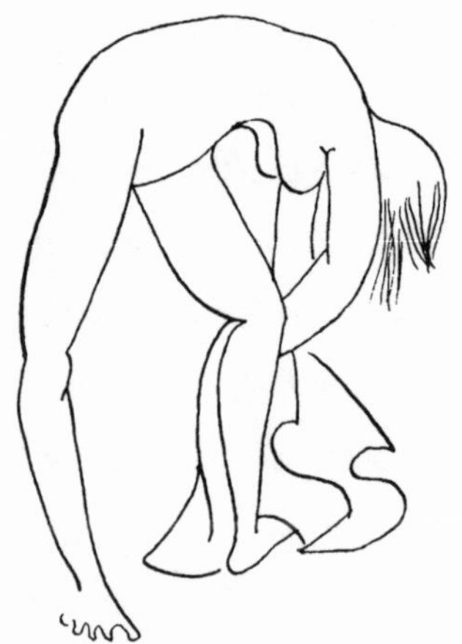

Pros

- *If a CT scan, MRI or myleogram have proven negative, but the doctor still suspects a herniated disc, this will usually make a positive diagnosis.*

Cons

- *No anesthetic is used and this is a painful test. The nature of the pain produced helps determine the problem.*
- *One patient recently reported, "If the discs are okay then you're okay, but if there is anything wrong, you'll be in pain."*

BONE SCAN

An injection of a radioactive substance is injected into your veins. A few hours later, a geiger counter is used to distinguish concentrations of dye. Dye concentrates in new injury sites. Old scar tissue doesn't absorb dye. Thus, doctors can tell if a fracture is old or new. It shows infections, tumors, arthritis of the spine, and can detect cancer.

Pros

- *Approved by the FDA for children. Less radiation than x-rays.*

Cons

- *The four hour test requires that you lay on your stomach for four hours. This is not the recommended postition for back patients.*

❍ EPIDURNAL VENOGRAM

Radiopaque fluid is injected into the groin and flows into the veins in the back. If a disc is bulging enough to compress a nerve root, it is usually bulging enough to compress a vein as well. Not used much since the CT scans, MRI's and discograms.

Pros

- ◇ *It has the least discomfort of almost any test involving an injection. Cheaper than CT scans and MRI's.*

Cons

- ◇ *It is an x-ray test that requires a highly skilled interpreter. CT scans and MRI's can show this area much more clearly.*

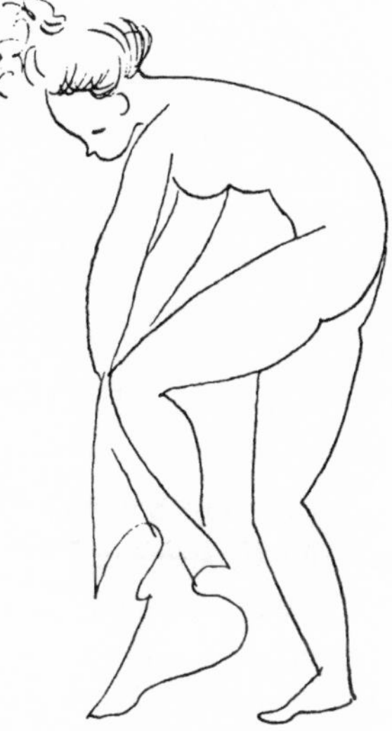

❍ EPIDURAGRAM

Radiopaque material is injected outside the sac (rather than inside like a myleogram), and is allowed to flow around the dura, to outline any bulging discs.

Pros

- ◇ *Because there is more fluid injected, and it can travel around a greater area, many medical people feel it offers a better chance of detecting a disc protrusion. It has the advantage of not irritating the inner lining of the sac, one of the greatest complications of a myleogram.*

Cons

- ◇ *It is an x-ray test. CT scans and MRI's can show this much more clearly.*

❍ NERVE ROOT INJECTION

§ *Make sure if you're sitting on a couch that you sit up straight and fill in the back with throw pillows.*

Local anesthetic and radiopaque liquid are mixed together and injected around the suspected root to determine which nerve root is to blame for an area of leg pain. The anesthetic removes all feeling from that branch. So if the pain ceases, that may mean that the trouble has been located.

Pros

- ◇ *Pain may temporarily cease because of the local anesthetic.*

Cons

- *Imprecision – different adjacent nerve roots often overlap in function. Adjoining nerve roots may be cited as the problem instead of the one causing the problems.*

❍ FACET INJECTION

Much the same idea as the nerve root injection but instead, the solution in injected into the facets to pinpoint which joint is to blame for facet pain.

Pros

- *Pain may temporarily cease because of the local anesthetic.*

Cons

- *Although more specific than the nerve root injections, the same overlap can occur. Also, neither the nerve root or facet injection test solves the problem of what to do next.*

"According to Swedish orthopedic surgeon Dr. Alf Nachemson, a pioneer in back pain research, slumping over a desk puts more stress on the disks and muscles of the lower back than any other posture."
– *Prevention Magazine*

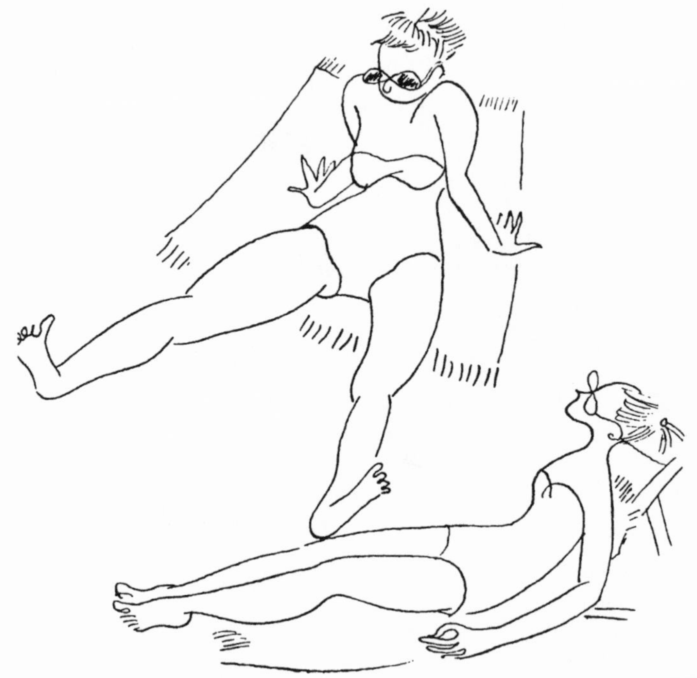

BACK SCHOOLS

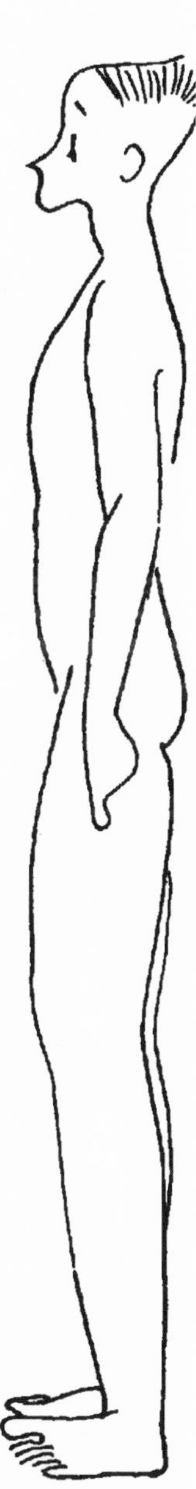

Back schools are currently a popular form of treatment for back pain, often recommended and sometimes required for patients considering surgery. These schools are often affiliated with hospitals but are also operated independently. The greatest advantage of a good back school is its multidisciplinary approach to the problem of back pain. Often there is a physician(s) who works closely with a team of physical therapists, occupational therapists, psychologists, and other support staff. Programs can be as thorough as 8 hours a day/5 days a week for a month. Each day is divided into time for videos and lectures, occupational therapy, psychology group, exercise classes, individual occupational or physical therapy time, relaxation technique class, and more exercise or pool classes. This kind of thorough back school program includes classes on every aspect of your back, of pain and how to successfully manage living with both. It can retrain even the worst offenders of bad posture and bad habits and can help reeducate you to participate in activities, from work to sports, that your back condition may have caused you to limit. Check with your insurance company to see if they cover back school programs.

❍ MENSENDIECK

"The schools are recommended for patients who do not need acute care but who must be educated about applying protective body mechanics to daily activities."
— Seymour Pedinoff, DO *et al, Patient Care*

The Mensendieck Method includes, but is not limited to these four major principles:

1. Proper alignment and balancing of all the various body parts during all activities.
2. Education of certain guiding principles to develop body sense and muscular awareness consciously.
3. Enlightenment as to the important relationship between mind and body and conversely, between body and mind.
4. The importance of active relaxation in the educational process.

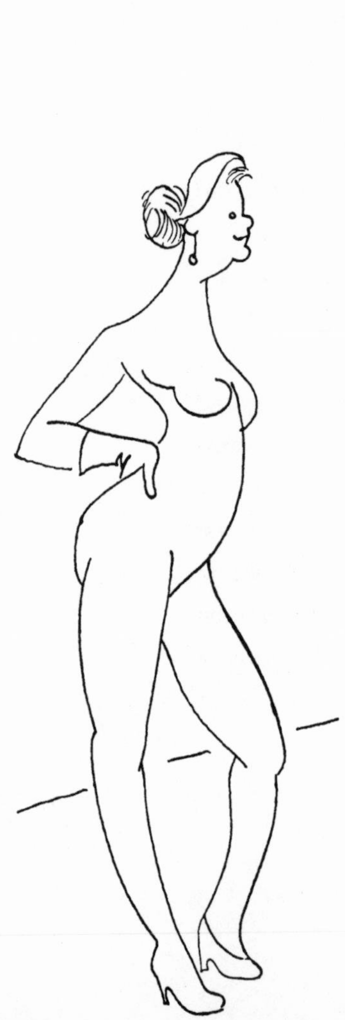

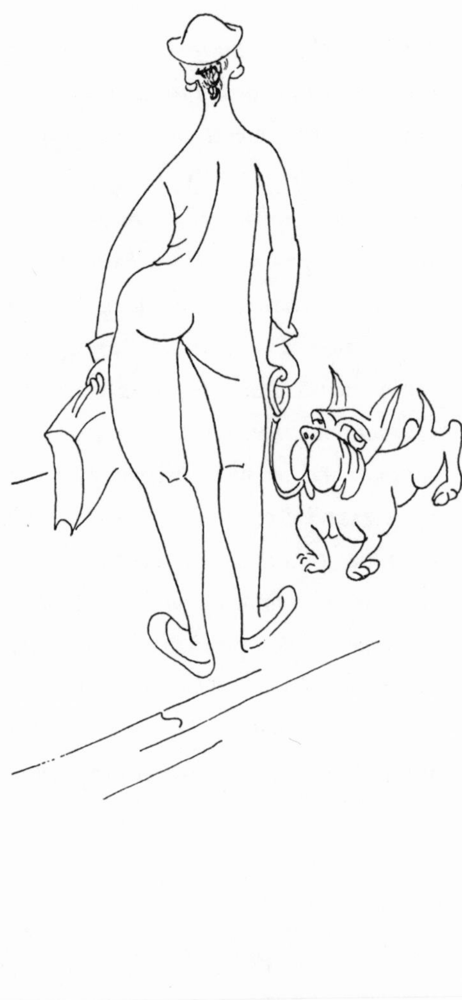

MENSENDIECK AND YOU

By Karen A. Perlroth

❍ PROPER POSTURE IS MORE IMPORTANT THAN YOU THINK!

No one is immune from back pain. Contrary to popular belief, most pain is not caused by sudden injury, but rather by the culmination of many small injuries which happen over a long period of time. Lack of exercise, weak muscles and years of misuse of the muscles of the back, abdomen, and elsewhere, and a general neglect of body mechanics can result in serious skeletal and muscular malfunction and pain. If you sit, stand, walk, run, sleep, exercise, and pick up and lift things incorrectly, your body will eventually protest. Living a sedentary life, being overweight, and/or suffering from stress are contributing factors. Warning signals are frequently given: stiff muscles, soreness, and loss of flexibility. Unfortunately, these signals are often ignored. A serious, stubborn, chronic back pain syndrome can be the result. . . sometimes for life.

Back pain isn't fun. It affects everything you do as well as affects everyone around you. Whether it is an ache when you get out of bed in the mornings, or pain in your back and leg while driving, or an all-out attack which puts you in bed, it is important to find out what's wrong. Identify a specialist and seek advice because serious disease needs to be ruled out. Do not allow this problem to get out of hand, or it will take you much longer to recover.

A popular European system which deals with proper body mechanics, posture and movement is called the Mensendieck System. Founded by a physician, it is based on sound scientific research in the field of kinesiology, the study of mechanics and anatomy in relation to human motion. This method consists of simple rules and can be

§ *Do all your errands in an orderly loop. Getting in and out of the car all the time wears on your back, and creates more time in the car sitting down.*

learned by anyone, at any age. It is part of the national health care systems in many Northern European countries and used as a preventive form of medicine and rehabilitation. It is gaining in popularity in the USA especially in the area surrounding Stanford University in California.

Mensendieck can teach you to direct and control your own muscle actions using conscious will power. It thus has mental as well as physical value. Eventually this will power, exercised over both the important act of breathing and over movement during all daily activities, will become habitual, providing increased energy, strength and a sense of well-being. Those participating in sports will find that they rapidly improve their techniques and stamina. Those who have no time for sports will find that they too will eventually look and feel better.

❍ POSTURE

Stand tall and well-balanced over the feet, with the body joints properly aligned.

A correct posture is less stressful than one which hangs, slumps and compresses the various joints and is the foundation for all subsequent Mensendieck work. A well-poised stance and gait will give you a sense of increased confidence and well-being. You will look and feel better, have more energy, and assume more control of your body and mind. Since no one is immune to occasional injury, it is wise to use good body mechanics and common sense on a day to day basis; you will recover and bounce back more quickly.

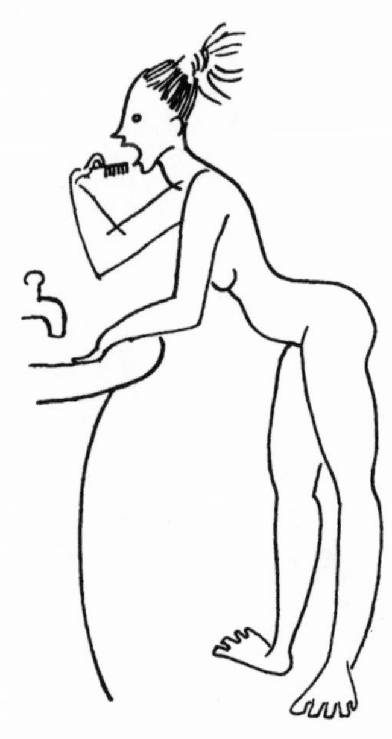

On the other hand, a lifetime of poor posture is asking for trouble. Your joints and bones will suffer, muscles and tissues will weaken, your circulation will become impaired, and your body will age more quickly. Moreover, if you don't sit or stand properly, how can you expect to walk, run or participate in athletics without hurting yourself eventually?

First and foremost you need your muscles for support and to keep your joints in proper alignment. When this happens, these same muscles can help move your frame with the least amount of stress. Good pelvic positioning using the appropriate muscle groups is also vital to maintaining a firm base in the middle of your body from which the spine can elongate, bend and straighten, and also support the weight of your head properly. When you have an erect, tall posture, your shoulders will be more relaxed and you will breathe more easily, enabling you to go through your daily activities in a more constructive and healthy way.

❍ WHEN BACK PAIN HITS

It is crucial that you know whether your pain is caused by muscle spasm, a joint problem, a bulging or ruptured disc, or an organic problem, especially if the pain is severe. If you notice weakness in your legs, or if you have trouble urinating, seek medical advice immediately. **Do not wait.** Seeking professional help to see you through the immediate, acute stage is both advisable and helpful. Severe pain will almost always mean some form of bedrest for a few days to take the stress and pressure off the affected area. Especially, if you suffer from a disk problem with radiating pain in your buttock, hip or leg, you need to take it very easy and go to bed for a few days until the acute radiating pain has disappeared. If you have pulled a muscle in your back you can be totally immobilized, however it does help if you try to stretch your spine very gently so that the spasm doesn't get worse. Usually a severe muscle spasm will respond to very gentle movement. Follow the directions about icing suggested in the First 48 Hours section of this book. But do only that which makes you feel better. Don't stay in bed for more than three days unless you suffer from severe leg pain or when your physician advises you to rest longer; because, in bed, your whole system weakens, your joints stiffen due to the lack of circulation and you could get blood clots in your legs.

§ *If your couch is foam, or starting to sag, you may want to put a board under the cushions.*

❍ WHAT TO DO WHEN YOU NEED BEDREST

The position you are probably most comfortable in is on your side. If you have sciatica pain in one leg you will most likely prefer lying on the opposite side. Use many pillows: place one against your abdomen so that you feel that it supports your back. Draw up your upper leg and place that also on a pillow. Your lower leg can be extended a little or bent whichever you prefer. Sometimes it helps to draw up both legs and place a pillow between the thighs. But in this position the circulation in your legs may become impaired. Sometimes placing the tiniest of pillows under your waist (still in sidelying) can bring relief. What is important is finding a position which is not painful. If you can change once in a while to a position on your back, then place one or more pillows under your knees. Lying on your back is not as

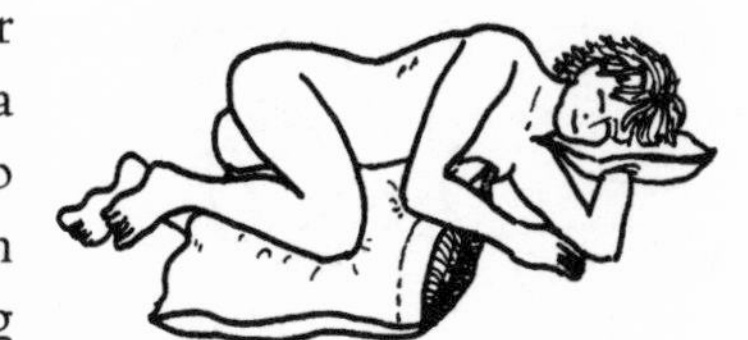

good a position as the sidelying because the back muscles tend to shorten. It is advisable to change positions once in a while, however.

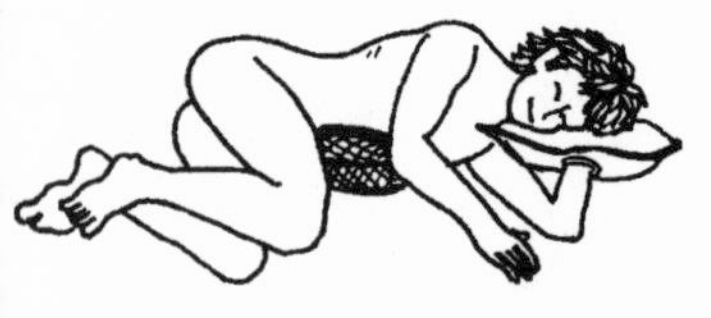

It is generally better to sleep on your side because your back muscles can relax more in this position. In sidelying, it is very important to always have a small pillow against your abdomen, (even after you recover) because this gives your back a chance to relax and stretch while sleeping or resting. This pillow will also prevent you from sleeping on your stomach which is very harmful because the lower back muscles tighten and cause hyperextension (hollowing) in your back while sleeping. It is also **not** good to sleep on your back always with a pillow under your knees because this will cause a shortening of the muscles behind them (hamstrings).

❍ SIMPLE EXERCISES YOU CAN DO LYING ON YOUR SIDE IN BED

In order to relieve back pain, attention *must* be paid both to correct breathing technique and correct body mechanics. In order to do so, follow steps 1 through 4 in order:

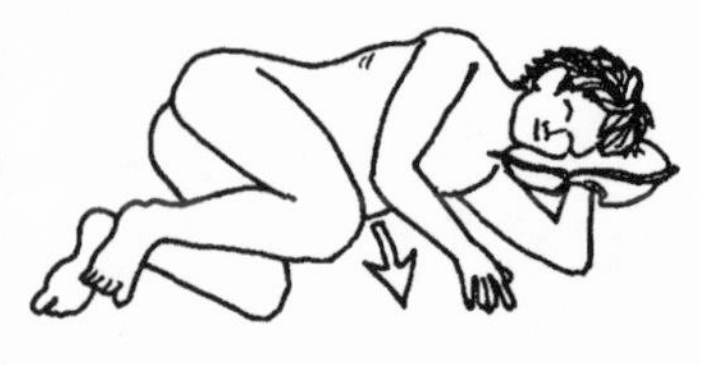

1. Breathe in gently through your nose. (Pretend you smell a pleasant aroma; breathe deeply, allowing your ribcage to expand fully.) Now breathe out again gently through an open mouth. Do not purse your lips or make noises while exhaling. Remain relaxed in the rest of your body. Pause for a brief second after you breathe in or out. This will slow your breathing and will assist you to relax. Repeat several times very slowly.
2. Breathe in again gently through your nose, but now concentrate on your abdomen and allow it to sag out by relaxing your abdominal wall. It helps at first to place your hand on your abdomen so that you can actually push against it when inhaling. On exhaling (out through your mouth) draw the abdominal wall in gently. You will now be contracting your abdominal muscles. Some of you may never have experienced this proper contraction. Continue to do this a few times and get used to this feeling. When your abdomen expands outward, your ribcage will expand less. it is important to realize that this is an abdominal breathing exercise, and not to be confused with normal breathing which should take place in the ribcage.

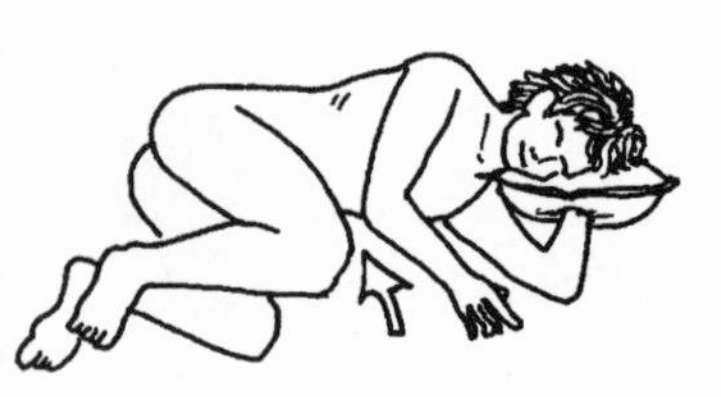

When you take air in, your lungs and chest expand. If you have your abdomen relaxed it will also expand. If you were to keep your abdomen drawn in tightly only your chest would expand. Think about it for a moment and experiment. You may have been in the habit of sucking in your abdomen while inhaling and releasing it again on exhalation. This is incorrect. Your abdominal wall can contract most effectively while exhaling because your chest and abdominal cavity become smaller when you breathe out, thus the muscles can shorten more effectively. Eventually your lower abdominal wall should be drawn in at all times except when you relax. Normal breathing occurs with chest expansion while the lower abdomen remains contracted.

"Good backs are those that don't hurt and bad backs are those that hurt all or part of the time."
— Jeanne Rose, *Herbs and Things*

Do not rush through this process. It is vital that you understand proper abdominal muscle contraction because you will need to make it part of all your daily movements. Good strong abdominals will help support your back in ways you have never thought of before. Drawing or pulling inward the whole abdominal wall is the proper contraction you need. It is not enough to bear down and tighten the muscles without drawing them in. Since you have nothing else to do but lie in bed you can spend plenty of time on this. It will be time well spent! Try it a few more times before you go to the next exercise. For those of you who are pregnant, it is vital that you learn to support your baby with a tight abdominal wall. You will lessen the strain on your lower back and hip joints considerably, prevent stretch marks, and improve your overall posture. Tightening your abdominal muscles firmly will not hurt the baby! After delivery you can regain your figure more rapidly.

3. Breathe in again gently through your nose, allowing your abdomen to sag. Pause a second and then, while exhaling, start drawing in your abdominal wall and contract or pinch your buttock muscles together also. Do this a few times very slowly, then relax. If you experience pain, tighten less firmly. Experiment a few times, but keep it slow and relax often. If it feels OK you can go to the next step.

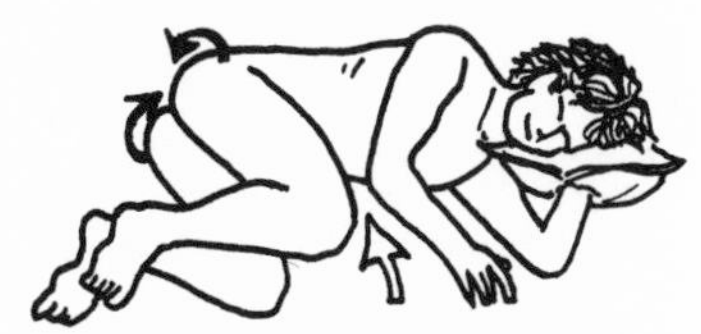

4. Same as above, but when you pinch your buttocks together also tuck under a bit, as though you have a tail and want to pull it under you. Then slowly while inhaling release both abdominals and buttocks. Do this gently over and over again. Never hold the contraction, just allow movement to occur in your lower back as you contract exhaling, and release while inhaling. If you have a bad spasm in your back muscles this may hurt a little or

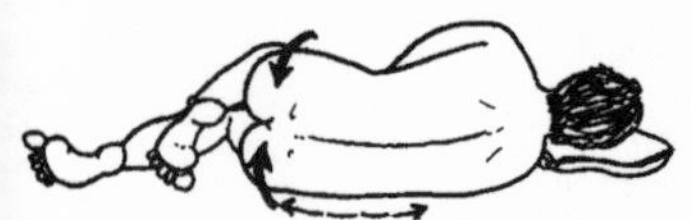

a lot because while you tuck you will find that your back will round out a bit. Muscle spasm is caused by your body's own natural immobilization process to prevent further injury to that area. It takes time and patience to break up this spasm. The shortened muscles have to be stretched gently. Tightening them and then releasing them again, over and over again, is what will break up the spasm eventually. Blood will be able to flow more easily into the muscles and this also helps to break it up. Consult your physician about proper medication to take if needed. If you have radiating pain your hip, buttocks or leg, you may have to be even more careful and gentle. Contract and move only as much as is comfortable.

○ SIMPLE EXERCISES YOU CAN DO LYING ON YOUR BACK WITH THE KNEES DRAWN UP

If you are comfortable lying on your back, you may now turn from your side to your back, but you first must pull in your abdominal wall again. Keep it tightly drawn in while you are turning over. In this manner there should not be any pull on your back. When lying on your back, be sure to keep your knees drawn up with the feet flat on the mattress. Your back should be in touch with the mattress. Now you can do the same exercises as you did lying on your side.

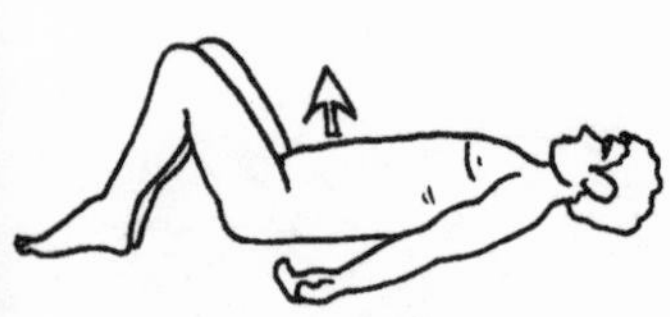

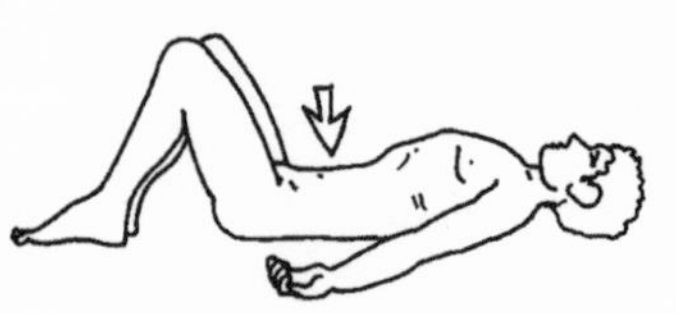

1. Breathing in and out, release and contract your abdominals again. This time when you breathe in (smell that aroma again and breathe in through your nose) expand the chest and abdomen upwards. Pause a second, and, then, when you breathe out through an open, relaxed mouth, draw abdominal muscles tightly inward and flatten your stomach. Place a hand on the lower abdomen so that you can make sure that you are drawing inward and not pushing upwards, a common mistake made in the beginning. Draw inward and down towards your inner spine. Repeat about 5 times, then rela::. If your back hurts then you have pushed your spine down too hard. Your lower back should be brought flat against the mattress.
2. Now, when tightening the abdominal muscles, also involve your buttock muscles by contracting them together and under while exhaling. While breathing in relax fully abdomen and buttocks. Do not hold the contraction at any time. Breathe slowly and contract exhaling and release inhaling. You will

find that you will begin to move your pelvis very gently forward and back. Your abdomen and buttocks releasing will mean that your lower back may arch a bit off the mattress. This is fine, because when you contract again your lower back will come back towards the mattress. When your lower back arches slightly it means that the muscles in the back contract, when your back is lowered again the muscles are forced to stretch. This creates a healthy exchange between relaxation and contraction which will aid the circulation and will also make you more aware of the muscles responsible for moving your pelvis. These muscle groups are very important in giving support to the body when standing and moving around, so none of this is wasted time. Do a few of these every 15 minutes or so while you are resting in bed.

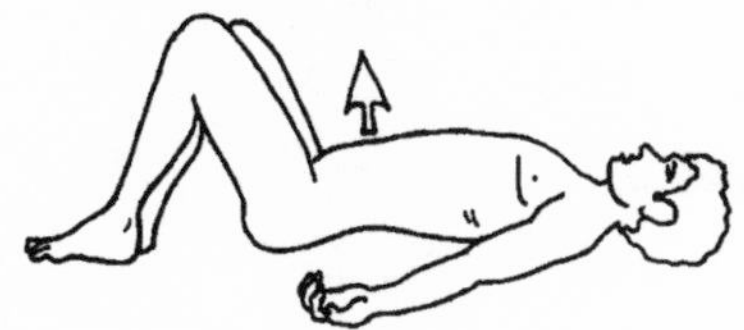

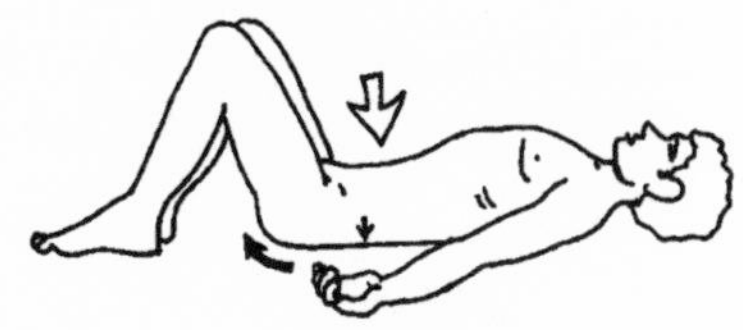

3. Sometimes it feels great to draw your knees up from the mattress. Clasp your hands together around the top of your knees and rock them **very gently**. Do not hold and pull, just rock the knees a little. In order to raise a knee upward you want to make sure that you contract your abdominal muscles first, because you have to stabilize your back and pelvis. If you don't do this your back will probably also hurt more. Follow these directions carefully. If you are in acute pain, you will have to wait a day or two:
   a. Inhaling, draw in your abdomen and buttocks, making sure the lower back is firmly against the mattress, and raise one bent knee off the bed until it is comfortably up. Exhaling again, tighten the abdomen inward and downward (don't let it pop up) and now also contract the buttocks together and lower the foot back down (keeping the knee bent) **all the time keeping you back firmly against the mattress**. Your pelvis may not move and your lower back may not arch while the leg is being raised or lowered. This is crucial for the stabilization process to take place. You need to fix your pelvis in a stable position from which you can teach yourself to raise one knee up and down. Later when you feel stronger and your pain has gone, you can raise a straight leg up and down using the same technique. **Never ever** raise both extended legs up and down at the same

time!! Repeat the same knee twice more before repeating with the other knee 3 times. Then relax.

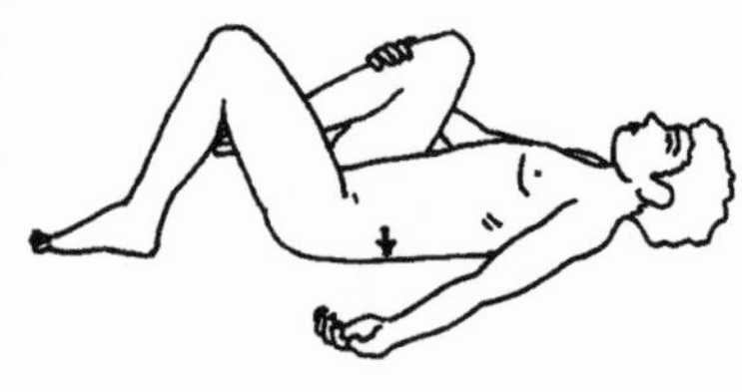

b. To raise both knees up, do not lift them simultaneously. After you have raised one knee up, hold on to it with one hand. Breathe in, and then, when breathing out, pull gently a little on the knee which is already up and then raise your other knee up as well. Fold your hands together and grab both knees. Now you may rock the knees very carefully. Do not pull and hold, but rather rock the knees carefully. Using the same method of breathing and contracting, lower the first leg you brought up (keeping it bent). Holding on to the other knee is helpful in keeping your pelvis stabilized. Then lower the other knee. When the second leg lifts up or when it is lowered, make sure that your back remains flat against the bed, and that the abdominal wall does not pop up (place other hand on your abdomen to test). Many people cannot accomplish this without their abdomens protruding and arching their backs while tilting their pelvis forward. If you suffer from severe buttock or leg pain, you may experience pain when both knees are up or when you rock. If that is the case, skip this until a later time. Do not do this if it hurts. Instead, try it again in a day or so.

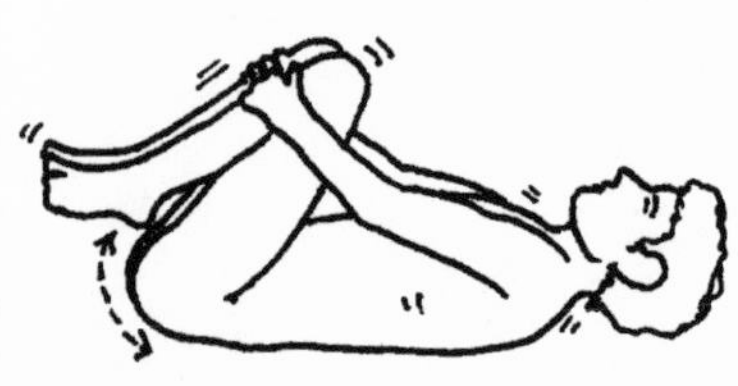

c. When extending your knees while lying on your back, you use the same stabilization practice. Do one leg a few times while the other remains bent with the foot on the mattress: while exhaling, tighten abdomen and buttocks while bringing your lower back firmly against the mattress. Keeping this position straighten your knee slowly keeping the heel in touch with the mattress. Only when the knee is almost straight may you relax the hold on the buttocks and abdomen! To bend the knee back up again, inhale slowly first, then upon exhaling, tighten abdomen and buttocks again while positioning your pelvis firmly by lowering the small of the back again against the mattress. Your knee will start bending again automatically and while keeping the heel in contact with the mattress, draw the knee back up again gently. Relax the hold around your pelvis only when the knee is fully drawn up. Practice this a few times with each

§ *At theatres, nightclubs, and school auditorium-type functions, inflatable back cushions can be brought along. I use a purse for lower back support when I know I won't be there too long – jackets that can be folded up work better than nothing.*

leg until you understand this process. At the end, draw each knee up separately (feet off the mattress) and, placing your hands around your knees, rock them again gently.

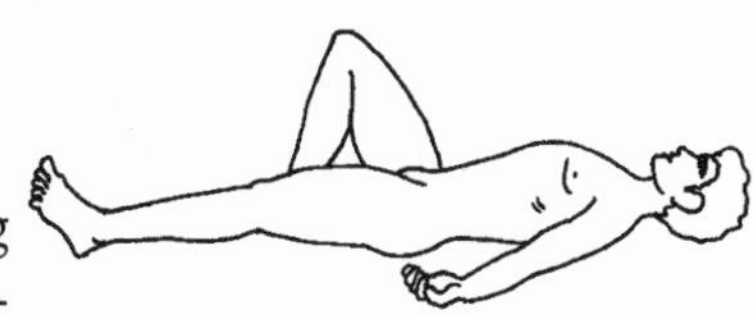

When you begin to understand this process of breathing, contracting and pelvic stabilizing, your back will begin to feel better as your muscles strengthen. You can apply this technique to everything you do. When you roll over, when you rise up, when you sit down, when you have to pick up or put down something, *etc.* Even before you sneeze or cough you can prepare yourself. Get used to contracting while changing positions. Eventually your abdominal wall should always be drawn in, except when relaxing or sleeping.

❍ SIMPLE EXERCISES ON HANDS AND KNEES

Another position in bed which can bring relief is on your hands and knees. Turn over to your side (exhale and draw your abdomen in and hold it while moving) and push yourself up until you are on all fours on the bed: *i.e.* your hands should be under your shoulder joints, your knees under your hip joints. Flatten your back, do not arch or hollow it. Draw your shoulder blades down and together a bit. Do not arch your neck by looking forward. Your neck should be an extension of your straight spine. This position can bring relief to your back by doing various gentle movements

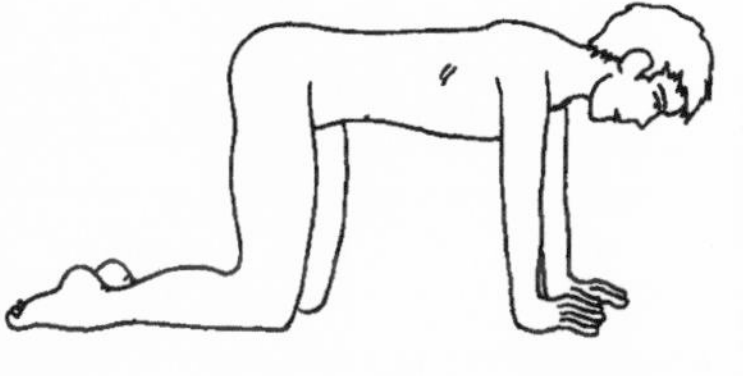

1. Inhaling, release all tension in your abdomen and allow it to sag down. Keep your back still. Exhaling, draw in the abdominal muscles firmly. Start the contraction in the lower abdomen, rather than the upper half. Inhaling again, release the tension slowly in your abdominal muscles, but do not allow your back to sag. It may not move. Repeat 5 times.
2. Inhaling, release all tension in your abdomen and allow it to sag down. Exhaling, draw in the abdomen and also tighten the buttock muscles gently together and under. Your lower back will begin to round slightly stretching the muscles in your back (tailbone down). Be careful and see how it feels. Your head may bend down a little. Inhaling again, slowly release the tension in your abdomen and buttocks and allow your back to gently sag down a little (tailbone up). This sagging occurs because your pelvis will tilt forward in the hips when the abdomen and buttocks release. Your lower back muscles will

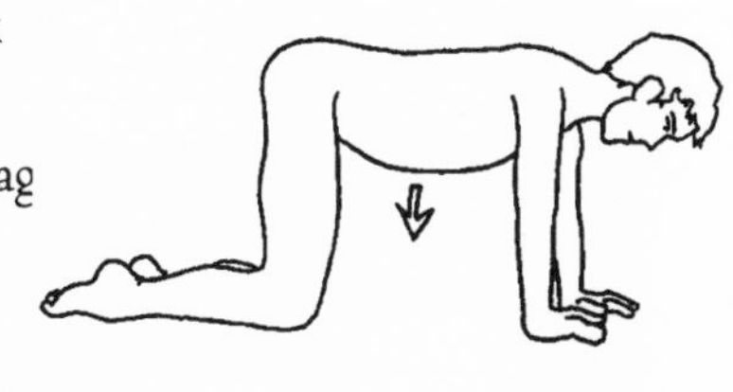

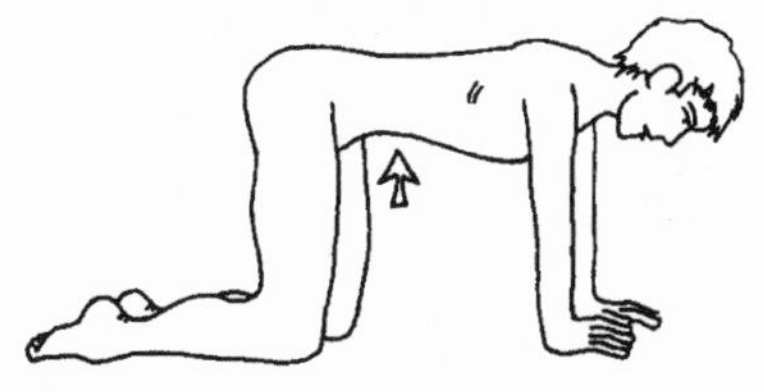

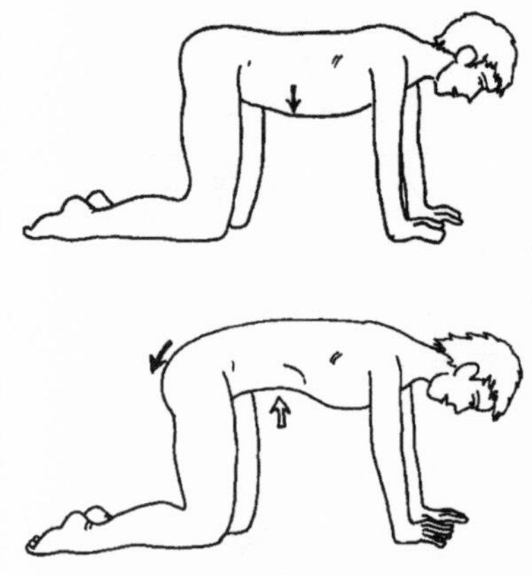

now contract. Keeping your shoulder blades drawn together a bit in the middle of your back is helpful. Do not have your shoulders drawn up to your ears, but rather bring them down towards your pelvis. Your head should come back to its original position, neck parallel to the bed. Repeat this gentle movement inhaling while releasing and arching the lower back ever so lightly, and exhaling while contracting and rounding your lower back ever so slightly again. Most probably this movement will give you some relief. If the spasm is severe, be very cautious. You may not be able to hollow your back at all. Do not worry, patience is needed.

3. When the lower back is rounded slightly (tailbone down) with your abdominal muscles drawn inward, exhaling, rock your body gently back a little, back and forth. See how that feels. Rock 4 or 5 times, then come back to the original position. Inhale, release abdomen and buttocks, sag, and then again exhaling, draw in, round your lower back ever so slightly,and repeat the rocking. Try to go further back each time. Eventually, depending on your own situation, you may be able to lie back with your buttocks on your heels, elbows sideways, and your forehead resting on the mattress, shoulders relaxed. When you can accomplish this, you can be sure that your situation is improving. (To come out of this position: lift your head up and simultaneously lift up with your elbows and move the upper body forward. When your head is between your hands, draw the shoulder blades together and straighten your elbows. Your back should be flat when you are back in the all-fours position.) To return to either sidelying or backlying, tighten your abdomen and buttocks. Repeat this rocking back and resting briefly with your forehead on the mattress and lifting up again a few times. Then return to your resting position on your side. Be sure to slowly turn until you are in the position you want to be in. Again, it helps a great deal to breathe out while contracting and moving.

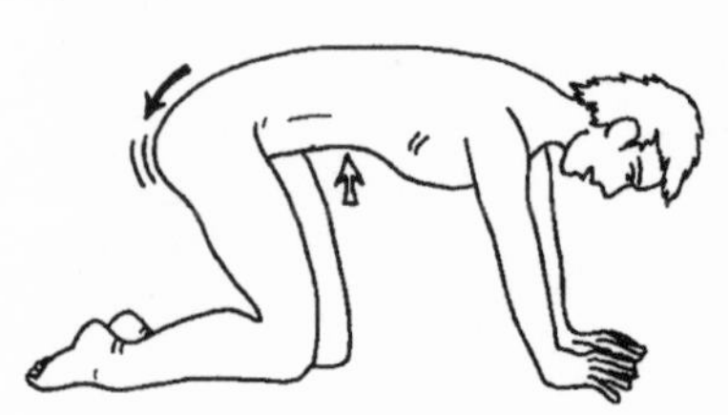

When you improve and you can get out of bed easily, your pain has subsided and your energy is slowly coming back, you should continue doing all of the exercises above. You may now do them on the floor on a rug or pad. This is preferred to lying in a bed. You want a good firm surface to exercise on. Continuing the exercises will strengthen the muscles and your awareness and

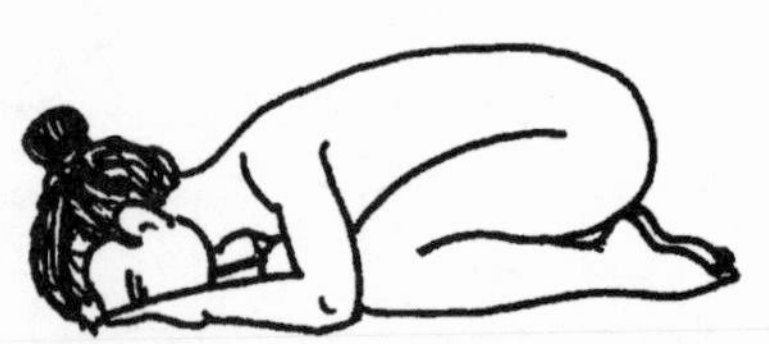

enable you to obtain improved upright posture faster. These exercises will also relieve any stress in your back. Make them a part of your life.

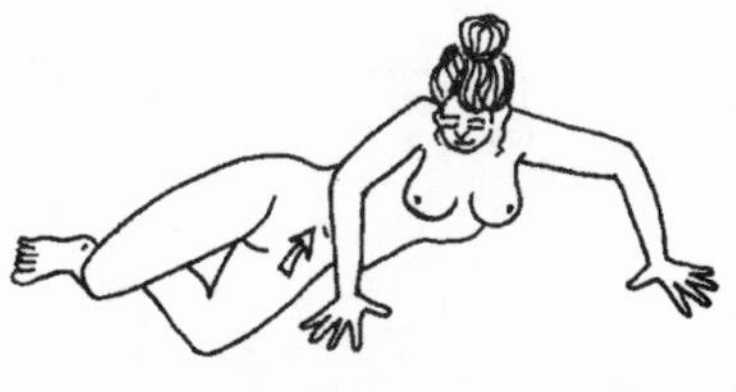

Getting up from the bed can be done with the least amount of pain and stress to your back if you apply all of the rules from the above exercises: From a sidelying position contract your abdominal wall inward, push yourself up from the mattress while bringing your legs over the side of the bed. It is best to position yourself slightly sideways on the edge of your bed. Place the leg closest to the bed forward a little (foot flat on the floor) while touching the mattress. The other leg should be placed back a little with the heel up an inch or two. Breathe in, and while breathing out tighten up abdominals and buttocks, bend forward a little if possible and push off with the hand closest to the bed. Your weight should have transferred to the front leg. It is very important that the rear heel remains elevated. This enables your pelvis to be in a safer, more stable and less stressful position. As you improve, you may need less and less support from your hand as you lift yourself off the bed. But especially in the beginning, if you are in severe pain, this is the least painful way to get out of bed, or up from a chair. The process for sitting down again is the same in reverse. Always keep the rear heel (from the foot placed back) elevated. This sounds complicated but it really isn't if you try it. **This position with one foot ahead of the other and the rear heel elevated makes all the difference in proper pelvic stabilization!**

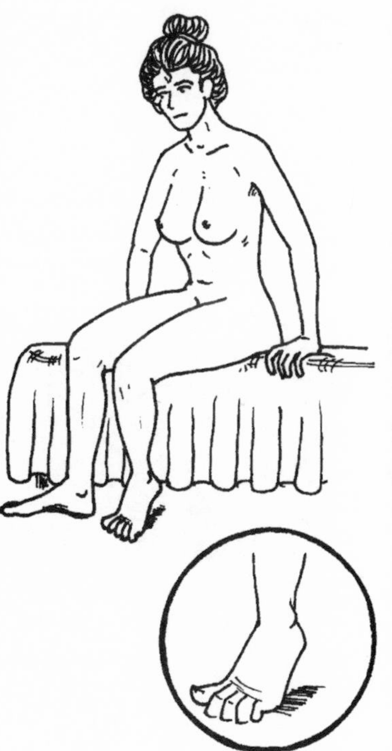

As you practice you will become more and more aware of how important this pelvic stabilization process is. Abdominal contraction exercises can be done in all different positions. For example:

❍ SITTING

Sitting at your desk, or at the dining room table, you can practice contraction exercises. Make sure that you are sitting tall on the bones at the bottom of your pelvis. If you are not sure where they are then place your hands, palms-up, under your bottom. Rock back and forth. The bones you feel are your sitting bones. It helps to place one foot forward flat on the floor. Your knee and ankle should be in right angles. Place the other foot back under the chair with the heel drawn up slightly. Draw in your abdominals firmly and keep them drawn in while you breathe in and out expanding the ribcage. You are now sup-

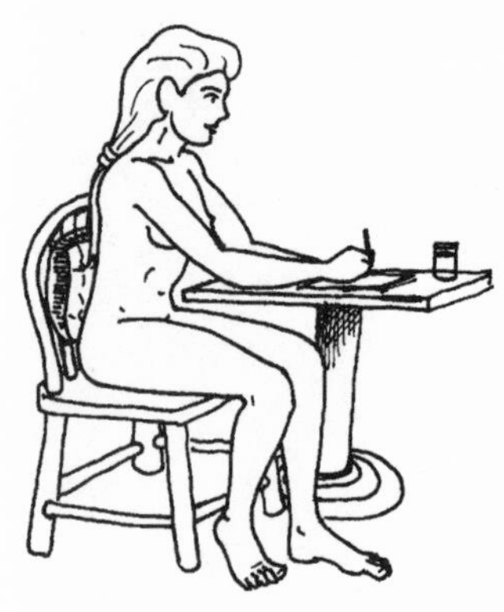

porting your back while sitting. This position is helpful when you have to eat or work at your desk or computer. Of course, it is vital that your back remains tall, that your shoulders are relaxed and down, with your shoulder blades drawn toward each other gently. You can accomplish this more easily by elevating your breastbone forward and upward. All of this takes practice and patience. You may, of course, sit deep back in the chair and support your back also with the back of the chair. If the seat is too deep, you may want to prop pillows behind you at first to give added support to your back while sitting, especially if you are in pain.

When you need to reach forward on the table or desk, be sure to tighten up again firmly while reaching. This action will support your back. For example, to reach your telephone, or to pick up something from the table or desk. If you do not tighten your abdominal muscles, your back has to support you.

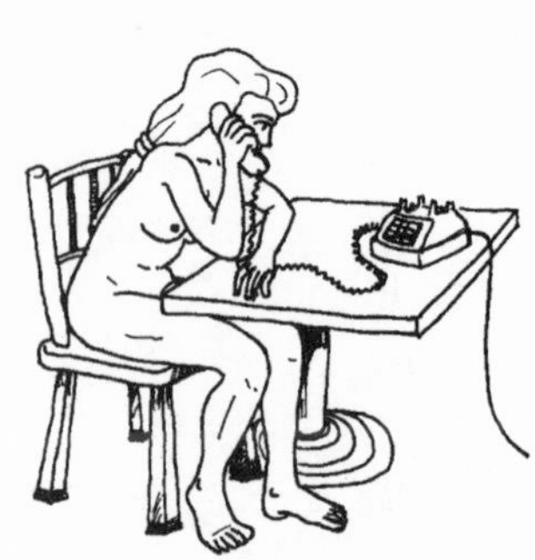

NOTE: Some of the newer designs in office chairs have a lever which tilts your seat forward. This is a fine position for your back only if you draw your abdomen in firmly and keep your spine straight. In this manner when you type, write or sew, your body is leaning forward a little thereby taking the stress off your back, shoulders and neck. If you have a kneeling chair, the same rules apply. If, however, you allow your lower back to sway (hollow), you will gradually cause damage to it. Many people have injured themselves with the kneeling chairs because no instruction was given how to use them properly. When used correctly they can be very beneficial. As a matter of fact, you can take any normal chair and tip it forward by placing a board or a hardcover book (2 inches in height) under the two rear legs of the chair. Using good body mechanics, this can bring a lot of relief. Remember this is only a position to use when you have to lean forward over your desk, computer keyboard or sewing machine. It is not a position to use for sitting straight, talking to people for example. A good office chair is well worth the investment. The back of the chair should support the whole back, not just the small of the back. Furthermore, the whole chair should also be able to tilt back and rock. This is a comfortable position for reading or talking on the telephone. You can even place your feet up on the desk.

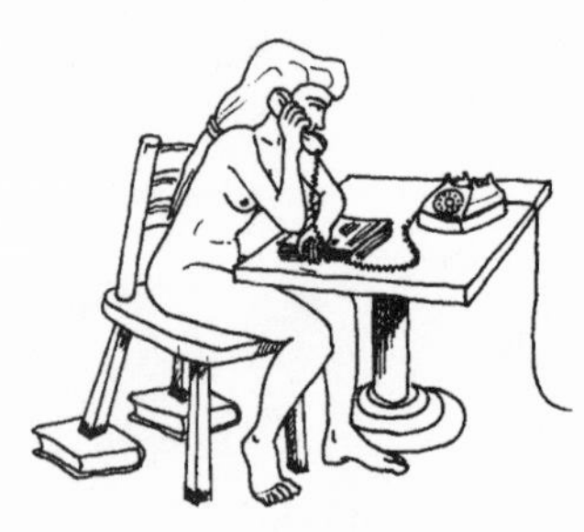

❍ STANDING

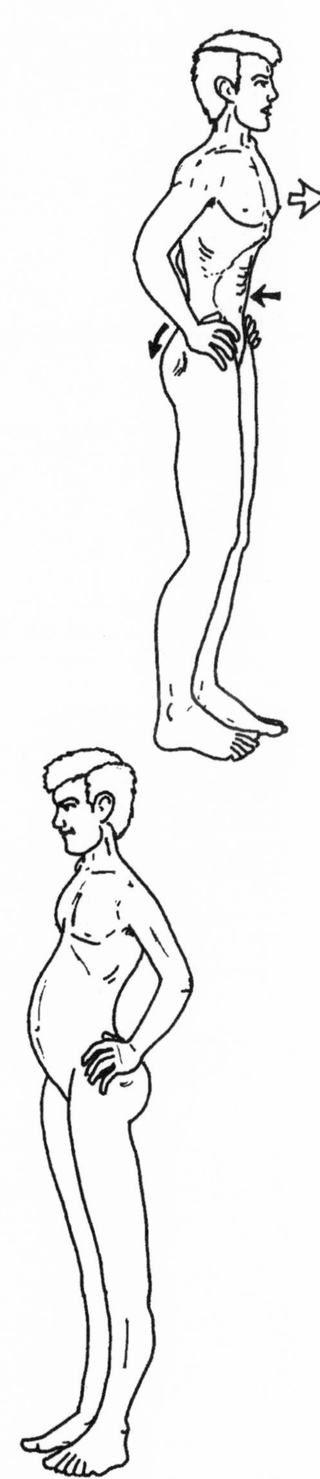

Standing tall will make a big difference! Observe your own posture in a big mirror. Placing your feet parallel and only a couple of inches apart is important. Do not toe out! Doing so invites back problems by tilting the pelvis forward and also causes your arches to drop (flat feet). You need good arches in your feet to act as shock absorbers for the rest of the body. If you are in the habit of toeing out, you can also get a myriad of other foot problems, such as painful bunions. Draw your buttocks together and tighten under a bit. This allows you to push the weight more forward toward the balls of the feet. (You may find that you always carried the weight of the body in the heels. This is very harmful because it throws off your posture and places a lot of strain in your lower back.) Contracting the abdominal muscles at the same time enables you to position your pelvis in an upright manner forming a firm base in the center of the body form which your spine can extend forwards and upwards.

Never lean back in the waist. Rather, with the abdomen drawn in and the buttock muscles contracted to keep your pelvis straight, lean a little forward in the waist and lift your breastbone up. This automatically improves the position of your head. Stretch up tall into your crown, with the chin down and in. Draw your shoulder blades down and gently together by contracting the muscles in the middle of your back. These muscles will assist you in keeping an upright, correct posture, while creating a very beneficial pull on the spine which maintains and increases bone density (prevents osteoporosis). This elongation of the spine upward decompresses the disks. If your upper back is slumped, all of your upper and middle back muscles hang slack, contributing not only to weak back muscles, but also weakened bone. A slumped forward posture also creates tension in your shoulders and neck which can result in headaches.

When you contract your buttock muscles, your knees will unlock and your large thigh muscles (the quadriceps) can contract and support the weight of the body upwards and out of the knees. Unlocking the knees is crucial, because it relieves stress in the knees. It prevents stretching of the knee ligaments, as well as compression of the knee cartilage, thus preventing unnecessary wear and tear in the knee joints. These are very easily harmed, and utmost care is needed so as to not hurry the natural aging process. Locking your knees also accentuates varicose veins and causes flabby thighs and hips. Contracting the buttocks while unlocking the knees causes the body weight to be pushed correctly forward towards the base of the big toes and the balls of the feet.

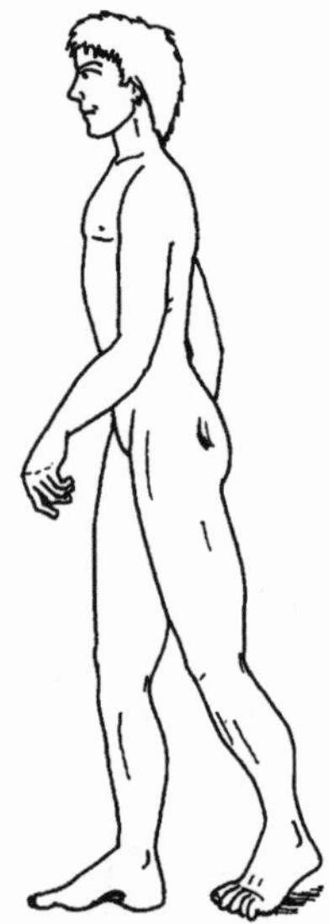

❍ WALKING

The posture for walking is very similar to the one you take for standing, but more so! Practice standing in good alignment. Tighten your abdomen firmly inward. Pelvis should be positioned upright. Lean slightly more forward in the waist, but keep the breastbone high with your chin in. Now pinch your buttock muscles a little harder. At this point, you will feel the body weight shifting more forward and you will want to start walking. Do so, and try to walk as lightly as possible, **always leading with your breast bone up high**. Your shoulders should be relaxed and down, with the shoulder blades drawn together gently a little. Your chin should stay down with a slight stretch in your neck upward to your crown.

Swing your arms gently in the shoulders, not in the elbows. Your feet should be pointing straight ahead at all times. If you were to stop suddenly, where do you feel you want to go? If your answer is "forward," you have passed the test. If, however, you feel (as you stop suddenly) that your bodyweight transfers backwards, then you have probably not leaned forward enough and your abdominal muscles were not drawn in enough. You were probably leading with your abdomen or with your legs. If you allow your abdomen to loosen, you will find yourself immediately leaning backwards in the waist. This causes a great deal of stress in the lower back and creates a heavy gait.

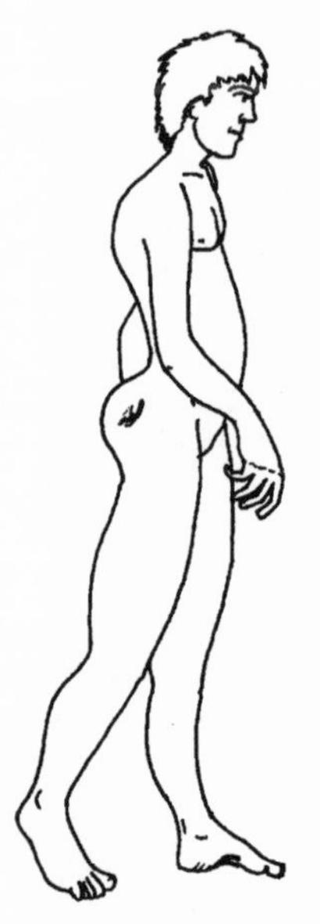

At first, you will find it difficult to walk with your buttocks pinched together a bit. Keep practicing because it will become easier quite rapidly and it will also help to firm up your thighs. Try stopping at times to see if your weight is forward enough.

If you run, or jog, it is even more important to lean forward in the waist with your abdomen held in tightly. You have to keep your feet absolutely straight ahead, otherwise you will create joint problems in the legs. Your back and neck should be in straight alignment, shoulders not tensed up, but relaxed and down, with a slight pull between the shoulder blades. Think "light" so that you will not pound on your joints excessively. Be sure to stretch before and afterward. For those of you who find jogging too stressful, keep in mind that a good brisk walk is easier on the body and can also provide a good cardiovascular workout with considerably less impact in the joints. People with back pain, with or without sciatica, should not jog or run. Walking or swimming (back stroke is best) would be easier for the back.

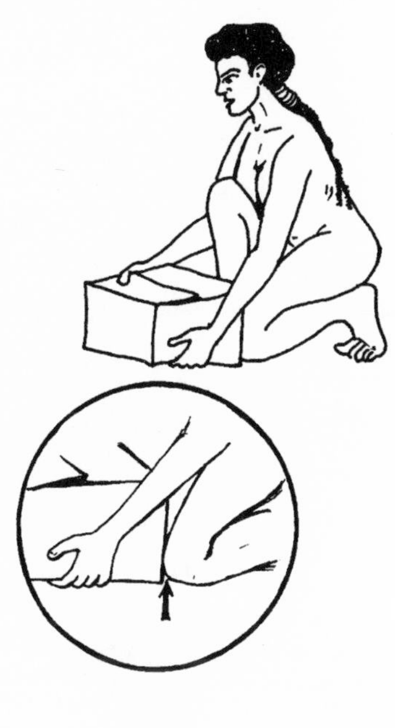

❍ BENDING AND LIFTING

The body has to be taught to work as a unit.

Place the feet parallel, one foot ahead of the other. (The feet are about 2-3 inches apart, with the toes of the rear foot lined up with the front heel.) Transfer the body weight towards the front foot. Keeping the heel of the front foot firmly on the floor, lean towards the base of the big toe. The heel of the rear foot is elevated about 2 inches. This position gives you a larger base on which to balance yourself properly. It is crucial that the rear heel remains up while bending, pushing, or lifting. The weight of the body must remain forward at all times. This enables you to keep the pelvis in the correct position throughout the movement.

Inhale first, then, while exhaling, contract abdominal and buttock muscles and fix your pelvis in a stable position. Keeping the weight in the front foot, carefully start bending your knees (thigh muscles contract properly if the buttocks are tightened) while keeping your pelvis stable with the abdomen drawn in. It is fine to bend the back forward slightly as long as you maintain tight control around your pelvis. This does not mean that your back collapses by allowing your breastbone to sink in. **Maintaining good elongation of the spine enables your long muscles to contract and support you. If you slump, these important muscles hang slack.** Trying to bend your knees while keeping your back absolutely straight does not work very well and often causes a swayback position (lower back arches too much), placing stress on the lower back.

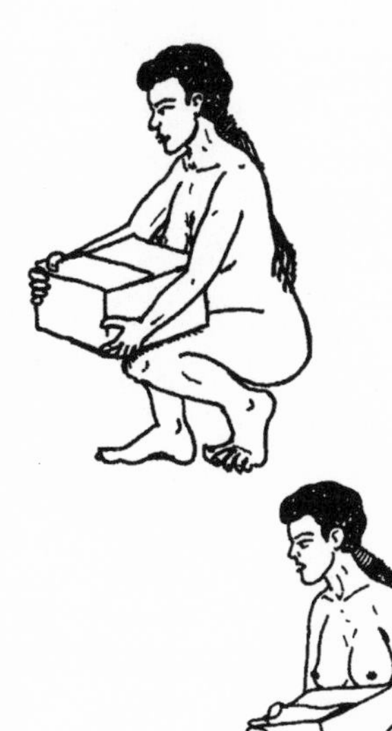

The combined contraction of buttocks, abdomen, and thigh muscles while bending the knees is vital. **Keep the bodyweight forward, toward the base of the big toes, at all times**, particularly when you straighten the knees upward again. If you allow the body weight to be brought backward into the heels, you will throw off your body alignment. Keep the rear heel elevated. Contracting your abdominal and buttock muscles while bending and straightening your knees creates good contraction of all your thigh and lower leg muscles and positions your pelvis in a safe, more stable, neutral position. Always keep your shoulders relaxed with the shoulder blades drawn downward and slightly together toward your spine. The neck stretches up

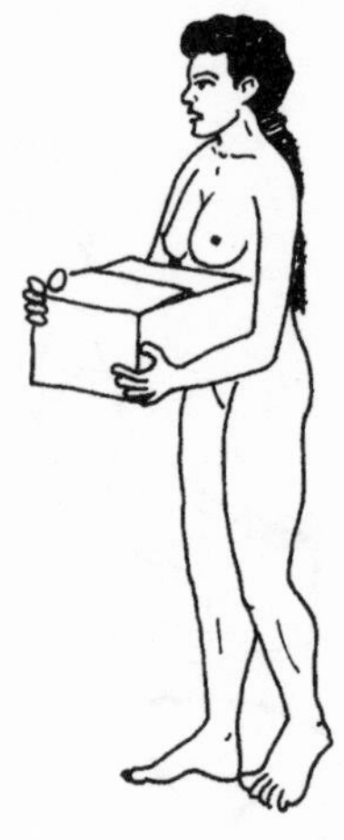

to your crown. The same technique is used for pulling or pushing. Use the body as a unit! **Exhaling, while drawing in the abdomen firmly when pushing, pulling, lifting, or reaching will protect your back. You will be amazed at how much lighter the object feels. Never hold your breath! This is dangerous.**

For those of you who have a serious back problem, you will have to find your own most comfortable position for bending and lifting. Some of you may want to bend more forward in the hip joints, others may not want to bend forward at all. No matter what, contracting buttocks firmly as described above will help you form a firm base in the center of the body. Place your stronger leg forward. If you have trouble bending the knees all the way down to the floor avoid placing anything on the floor! Get in the habit of placing things higher up, on a ledge. For those of you with children, get them to pick up their toys, socks and shoes. This is easier said than done, but it is possible.

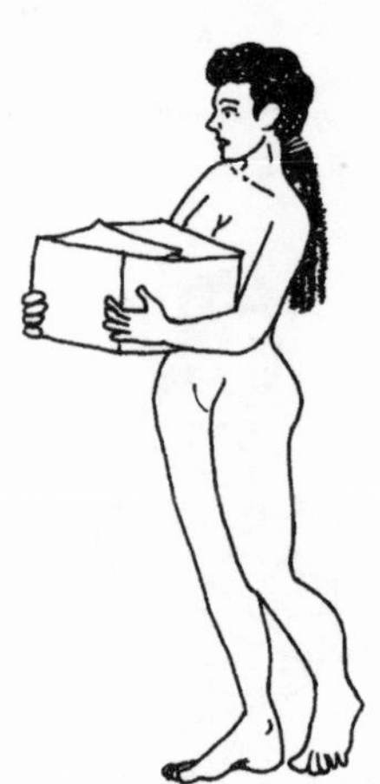

Brushing your teeth can often be very uncomfortable when your back is hurting. It actually helps to stand slightly at an angle at the sink. If you are right handed, stand with your right foot ahead and turned a little to the right. Your left foot should be parallel to the front foot with the heel slightly elevated. Since you are at an angle you can now bend with your knees parallel to the cabinet. Position your pelvis firmly with tight abdominals and buttocks. You can now bend safely over the sink. Reverse this process if you are left handed. If you need extra support, then lean on the opposite hand. Standing at an angle enables you to bend your knees more, thereby taking the stress off your back. Standing straight in front of the sink prevents you from bending your knees because they will hit the cabinet.

You will find that you can use this same principle in many other instances. Standing with one foot slightly ahead with the rear heel elevated enables good elongation of your spine and easier positioning of your pelvis. Standing at a slight angle can take the stress off your lower back. Taking groceries out of the trunk of your car would be a good example since the bumper would be in the way if you were to stand facing the car. But with the feet at a slight angle (always keep the weight in the front foot and the rear heel elevated), you can bend the knees quite far without interference from the bumper. Of course you may never twist while bending and picking things up. Many people get injured because they twist while pulling or lifting. This adds a great deal of internal pressure to your disks and can create a serious injury.

❍ SUMMARY

It takes patience, time, and some common sense to recover from a back injury. No matter how small or great an injury, allow this to be a learning experience. Teach yourself good body mechanics and improve your posture during all daily activities. If you have led a sedentary life, find some enjoyable, physical activity which you can do on a regular basis. However, working out once or twice a week aggressively, and then the rest of the time hanging sluggishly in your skeletal frame is not conducive to maintaining a healthy body. If you are an athlete, gain a new perspective: Why did you get injured? Were you pushing yourself too hard? Were you stretching enough before and after running? Were you using weight training equipment properly?

Gain a new positive awareness. Analyze your own movements and those of others. Learn from them and become healthier and stronger. Seek professional help if needed and listen to your own internal warnings if all is not well. Do not ignore them. Prevention goes a long way. The simple exercises which have been discussed here work. Combining a fitness program with these exercises using correct body mechanics and improved posture can keep you trim and healthy.

§ *Make your car seat comfortable. Either with a back cushion, or whole seat.*

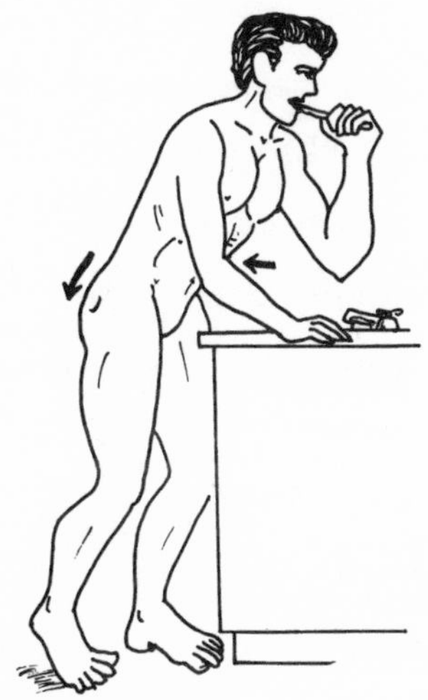

For information send a stamped, self-addressed envelope to:

Mensendieck Enterprises
P.O. Box 9450
Stanford, CA 94309-9450
Telephone 415-851-8184

Five videos are available, each with a 30 page booklet. Each video is $29.95 plus 8.25% California sales tax and $4.00 postage and handling. Send check or money order to Mensendieck Enterprises.

1. The Mensendieck System, Freedom from Back Pain
2. No Strain, No Pain, Back Fitness Program for Men
3. No Strain, No Pain, Back Fitness Program for Women
4. No Strain, No Pain, Back Fitness Program for Seniors
5. No Strain, No Pain, Back Fitness Program for Pregnancy and After Childbirth

The book *Mensendieck Your Posture* by Ellen Lagerwerff and Karen Perlroth, (Doubleday, 1973; revised by Aries Press, 1982) is available for $14.00 plus 8.25% California sales tax and $4.00 postage and handling.

§ *If you work at computers, make sure you have a chair that is ergonomically correct. Many companies that won't buy you a new chair will pay for a back cushion. Strongly recommended reading is Donkin's* Sitting On The Job. *Make sure that the middle of the screen is slightly below eye level.*

Karen A. Perlroth

Born in the Netherlands, and a graduate of the Mensendieck Institute in Amsterdam, Karen A. Perlroth is one of America's leading back therapists and educators. Since 1966, using this internationally acclaimed method, she has helped hundreds of men, women and young people overcome crippling back problems and resume normal, active lives.

She has taught at orthopedic, neuro-surgery and maternity clinics and rehabilitation centers, and at junior colleges and nursing schools. In addition, she is a consultant to construction firms, and has led many corporate seminars on Back Pain Prevention. She is also an ASPO/Lamaze Certified Childbirth Educator and has conducted many classes in Pre-Natal and Post-Partum care.

She is in private practice in Portola Valley, California, where she lives with her husband, a cardiologist and Professor of Medicine at Stanford University School of Medicine, and their children.

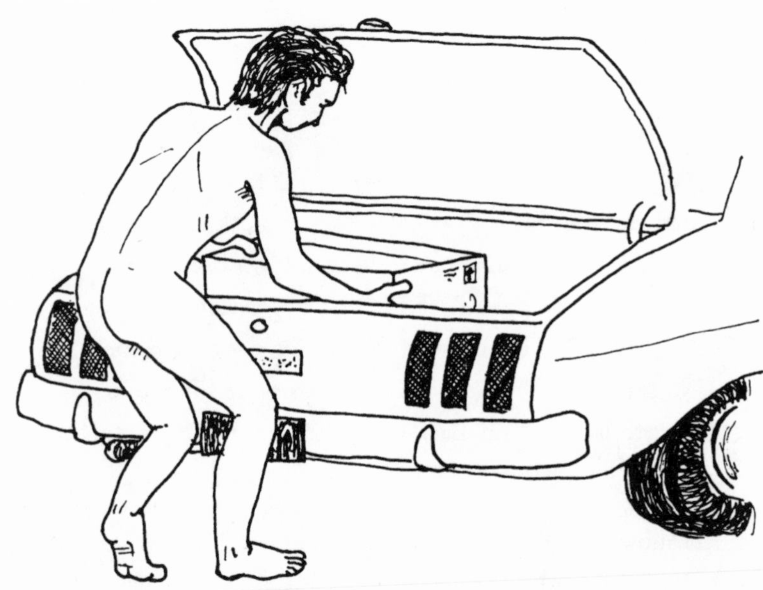

PAIN

What is pain?

We all know things that cause pain, but what exactly is pain? And why is something so common, so present, and so demanding, so hard to pin down?

"Research has shown that lack of exercise, driving for more than 20 minutes a day and cigarette smoking are all predictors for suffering back pain."
– Arthur White, *Shape*

The latest research on pain suggests that pain is experienced when certain nerves specifically oriented to intense, potentially harmful stimulation, nerves called "nociceptors," are excited. These nerves are part of the peripheral nervous system. The peripheral nerves communicate with the autonomic (automatic) nervous system, the reflexes, and other parts of the brain via neurotransmitters. Neurotransmitters are chemicals which bridge the gap between neurons, enabling the electrical impulse to pass from neuron to neuron along a path that leads to various sites in the spinal column and brain. Aspirin, for example, is now understood to act in part on nociceptive nerve endings.

There are a variety of physiological responses involved in pain. There is the reflex response, causing you to pull away from a hot stove, for example, before you become consciously aware of the burning sensation. Another response, the autonomic response, alters your body's vital functions, responding to a sense of emergency by releasing adrenaline, causing you to sweat or your blood pressure to rise. There is also an emotional response: fear, anger, annoyance, anxiety. Long term pain is suspected of causing nerve damage which creates hypersensitivity to pain, as well as causing emotional difficulties, since the emotions are an intrinsic part of the physiological response to pain.

In the search for ways to kill pain, researchers have tried to understand the many ways in which people experience pain, and not just how, but why it stops and starts. Thus far, the model with the best

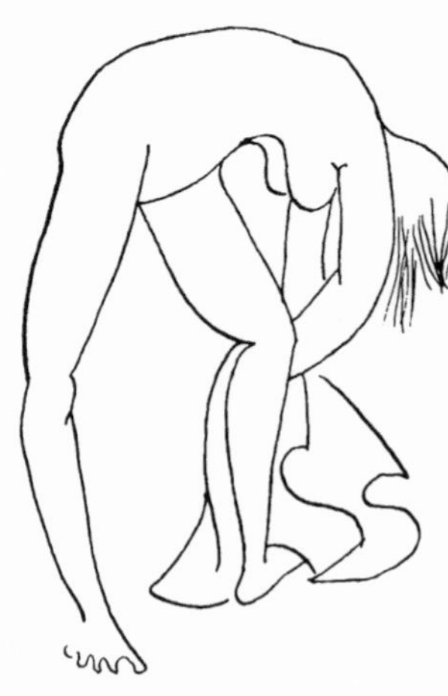

explanatory value is known as the "Gate Theory of Pain." Gate theory maintains that a certain number of neurons need to be stimulated to a certain level of activity in the peripheral nervous system before the "gate opens" and the pain message is sent along the neural pathways to the brain. According to this theory, there are also neurons present that can reduce activity in the initial group of neurons and thus prevent the "gate" from opening. For example, neurons that respond to non-painful contact like scratching or rubbing can perform this function.

Pain inhibition can also come from the other direction. The brain can secrete a type of neurotransmitter, one or more of a family of proteins known as Endorphins, that acts between the nerve cells to inhibit the pain impulse from passing from one nerve cell to another. Endorphins, which are structurally similar to opiates (morphine, heroin, *etc.*), vary in their strength and longevity. One, Dynorphin, is said to be ten times stronger than morphine. Chronic pain sufferers have been found to have lower levels of endorphins in their spinal fluid than non-chronic pain sufferers. There is not, however, an easy solution to raising these levels. Some endorphins break down more quickly than others and, like the opiates they resemble, they can be "addictive" or generate tolerance (reduced effectiveness of the same quantity).

Endorphin production has been connected (with varying degrees of scientific precision) to chocolate, laughter, exercise, love and spicy food. It is also suspected of being the mechanism at work in the Placebo Effect. Placebos, used as controls in experiments on the effects of new medications, consistently show an effectiveness rate of 30-40%. In other words, approximately one-third of all subjects given a placebo will manifest the desired result. In terms of pain, this effect is believed to be, at least in part, the result of the activation of the body's own pain killing system, a belief confirmed by the ability of an endorphin-inactivating substance to cause pain to return. The precise mechanism of this activation is still largely unknown, but it is consistent with the observation that individuals with a positive outlook and trust in their recovery process heal more quickly than those who are anxious or depressed.

§ *Make sure that the back of your head is still supported by the car's headrest if you get a car seat that has a 2-part back support and an attached seat.*

All of this only confirms that yes, sometimes pain is "all in your head" but that, even when it's not, a hug, a truffle, or a good laugh might be worth a try.

MULTIDISCIPLINARY CARE

Pain Management Programs for Low Back Disorders

by Hubert L. Rosomoff, MD and Renee Steele-Rosomoff, BSN

Thirty percent of our population suffers from chronic pain at a cost of 70 billion dollars annually. One third of these suffer from chronic low back pain which represents the single most costly health problem. Unfortunately, pain management programs are considered as courts of last resort where the patient is referred when all diagnostic and therapeutic efforts have been exhausted. Often, that patient is viewed as having a behavioral disorder in which there is little or no organic basis for the symptoms.

Presently, only four percent of patients in the USA with chronic pain are treated by pain management programs. The goals of an optimum program should be to:

1. Achieve a high level of function.
2. Reduce or eliminate pain and medication intake.
3. Teach prevention of reinjury or exacerbation.
4. Teach techniques to treat reoccurrence of pain.
5. Eliminate dependence on the health care system.
6. Enable patients to return to full avocational and vocational activities and
7. Achieve optimum wellness and quality of life.

The pain patient is extremely complex with physical, behavioral, vocational and psychosocial issues requiring a coordinated, integrated, goal-

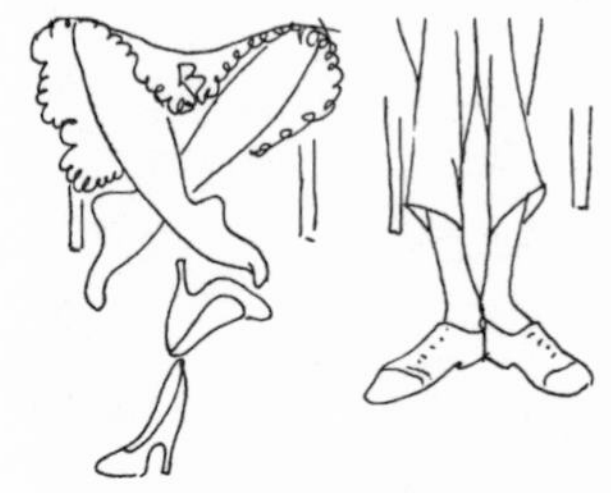

oriented multidisciplinary team approach. An autonomous inpatient setting, exclusively for the care of these patients, along with a contiguous outpatient setting are required in order to maintain a controlled setting. The intensity of service should provide an aggregate of basic, therapeutic and training services for six or more hours per day, five or six days a week, continuously for a month. Such a program should provide management of behavioral disorders, patient education, and daily therapy from physical medicine and other health care delivery disciplines, like rehabilitation nursing, and vocational counseling for job placement. Not to be overlooked are ergonomists who study human performance and environmental design. The medical staff must be available on a 24 hour basis, and daily visits and regular conferences in which all the health care deliverers participate are required.

During the developments of the University of Miami Comprehensive Pain and Rehabilitation Center, the program was a component of the neurological Surgery Department which did treat a large number of low back disorders. Some of the more complicated and difficult cases, such as those undergoing "salvage surgery," were put into the program as a post-operative rehabilitation effort. When this was found to enhance the outcome of the surgical results, patients were placed in the pain management program as a pre-conditioning phase to operation. The patients began to improve so rapidly that surgical indications could no longer be found. It became an inescapable conclusion that all patients with significant low back disorders leading to pain, disability and impairment, should be entered into the program before a final therapeutic decision was made of a surgical nature. As the years passed, the number of individuals going on to surgery decreased from five percent to two percent and, since 1981, has essentially been none. Patients with significant disorders are sent to the program whether or not they have surgical criteria.

"Burden-bearing thoughts can help create backache. If this is the case, a positive outlook should bring relief."
— *The Handbook of Alternatives to Chemical Medicine*

All patients with low back pain should be offered a multidisciplinary integrated type of program with the goal of pain and back rehabilitation for re-entry to work once the simple time honored approaches have failed. That is, if a patient has not responded to an initial short period of bed rest, followed by a physical medicine program aimed at restoration and conditioning, then no further time should be spent before moving on to a more aggressive level of management. Any initial competently applied regimen of conservative management should succeed in four to six weeks. If the problem continues beyond that period, then a more aggressive and comprehensive program should be sought. The major condition to the second level of management is behavioral review, including psychological assessment.

The development of the chronic pain syndrome is often the outcome of this bewildering variety of somatic pathology, emotional responses to the pain, physical responses, with the limitations imposed by repeated interventions and, further, feelings elicited by these changes. Since 85 percent of pain impulses project to visceral and behavioral brain, it is no surprise that emotional disorders appear in 95 percent of the patients.

The multidisciplinary team approach to the diagnosis and treatment of pain has evolved to overcome the difficulties single practitioners face in dealing with these naturally occurring or iatrogenically [treatment] induced problems. Patients are evaluated by a neurosurgeon, orthopedist, physiatrist, internist, psychiatrist, psychologist, physical therapist, occupational therapist, registered nurse, vocational counselor, when indicated, an ergonomist (industrial engineer) and other consultants as deemed necessary. A team dentist is utilized when temporomandibular joint syndrome (TMJ) must be ruled out.

The goal of the evaluating team is to identify all problems with which the patient presents and for which treatment is available. The problem list becomes the basis for the treating team care plan which is developed at the time of evaluation and which is modified and revised throughout the patient's stay. Chronic pain patients often report a long series of frustrating encounters with the medical profession where one consultation is held separate from another and information never seems to be brought together to form a coherent evaluation and treatment plan. The team approach obviates this problem.

The neurosurgeon, orthopedist and physiatrist are not only concerned with neurological status and skeletal stability, but they search for soft tissue causes of pain as well. These might include muscle spasm, tightness, trigger points, and weakness.

The team psychiatrist interviews each patient individually. Mental status is assessed, as well as the dynamics or problems of current significant relationships. The patient is asked to complete a pain history questionnaire, with details and development of the pain problem as well as attendant secondary problems and the degree to which daily activities are affected by the presence of the pain problem. Psychological testing is also administered; we use the Million Behavioral Health Inventory, an instrument which addresses various psychogenic

"Probably no more than 50% of patients can be given a precise diagnosis for their symptoms. In fact, the most common diagnoses rendered for LBP [Low Back Pain] are acute or chronic lumbosacral strain or sprain, fibrositis, and the general category of 'degenerative spinal disease.' In most instances, the diagnosis is a description of symptoms, rather than a specific pathologic diagnosis."

– John Frymoyer, MD

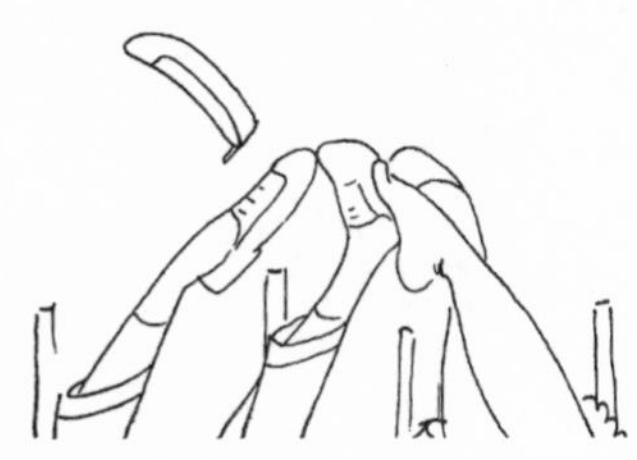

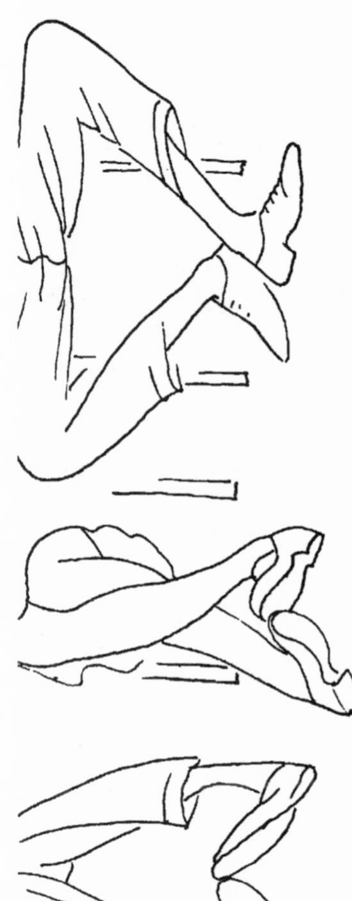

attitudes within the context of the personality traits of the individual. The significant other is also interviewed.

For entrance into the treatment phase of the program, patients must be medically stable, although it is not necessary that they be free of all disease processes. However, conditions such as uncontrolled diabetes or a serious cardiopulmonary impairment will create interference and prevent patient and staff from developing a continuous rehabilitation program. Behavioral disturbance is not a contraindication to entry, if the behavior is not disruptive to the community setting. Functional capacity is stressed with the goal of regaining normal activity levels rather than the reduction of pain. Detoxification is accomplished as treatment is initiated.

Treatment is carried out on a daily intensive inpatient or outpatient basis. Education and cognitive awareness are a significant component of the program. Efforts are made to create a high level of understanding of body processes and self-care. Lecture discussions are given throughout the program on a variety of topics such as body mechanics, anatomy, flare-ups and pacing, allowing clarification of questions that may have been a confused jumble of phrases and little understood medical jargon for a number of years. Emphasis is on adaptation of the human body, and its capacity to minimize the effects of pathology with proper management and training.

Physical therapy and reconditioning is an integral part of the program. Treatments include therapeutic exercises, heat, cold, transcutaneous electrical neural stimulation (TENS), and other modalities, as required. Modalities are generally used in the initial phases of treatment as palliative measures to ease initial discomfort when patients begin using muscles that have often not been used since the original pain problem occurred. Exercise programs include reconditioning, as well as specific exercises customized for the individual patient.

The occupational therapist has the responsibility for assessing the patient's standing, sitting and walking tolerances. These are the building blocks of many life activities, which the patient may or may not feel able to perform. Important is the evaluation of the patient's capacity to execute activities of daily life and the body mechanics of vocational and leisure time activities.

Behavioral modification is carried out in both the group and individual setting by the team psychologists with patients utilizing these milieus to share their feelings about themselves, their problems and the program, with their peers. Family groups and individual sessions for husbands and wives are also provided so that there is a carry-over of the team efforts into the home setting.

Vocational counseling, work conditioning and job readiness are essential elements for patients in the working age group so as to achieve and maintain successful outcome. The ergonomist is an integral member of the team and works very closely with the physical therapists, occupational therapists, vocational counselors and physicians to analyze the work place design and return to work requirements. This team constructs an individualized work conditioning program for the patient which simulates and incorporates most of the activities which will be required in the work setting. This enables the patient to return to work with confidence in his/her ability to perform and eliminate the potential for reinjury. Patients are expected to return to employment immediately following discharge. The majority of the patients completing the program have been able to return to previous employment, including heavy work, without limitations on their activities. The team will apply the same methodology to any leisure time activities like tennis, golf, skiing, karate, dancing, *etc.*

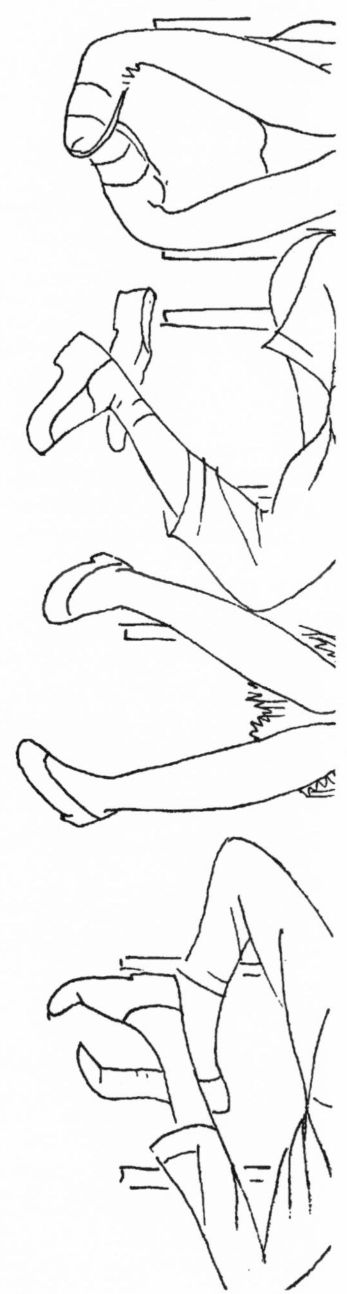

The final phase of treatment is discharge planning, completion of work conditioning activities and mastery of self-care and home maintenance program. Family involvement during this phase is essential to maintain the gains made and provide support. The significant other is encouraged to participate in the last few days of the treatment program. Rehabilitation specialists who are specifically trained in rehabilitation to make observations and manage this type of health care program may follow patients after discharge. This is extremely important when patients live at a distance. The ultimate goal is independence from the health care industry.

The basis of this program is the belief that low back injuries produce soft tissue trauma leading to pain, loss of function and disability. Herniated discs requiring surgical intervention are uncommon even when a neurological deficit is manifest, since soft tissue pathology can mimic these syndromes. Treatment requires aggressive management of behavioral aberrations, an expected concomitant of the painful state which are likewise reversible, including rapid detoxification from drug abuses. No single medical discipline can deal with these complex features, so multi-disciplinary action is required in a tightly integrated and supportive rehabilitative milieu.

Multidisciplinary management programs are less costly than surgery and its attendant losses from absenteeism, benefits paid and lack of productivity. Patients can be returned consistently to full function in an average of four weeks. Therefore, pain management programs have an important primary role in evaluation and treatment of low back pain, as well as an extended application to those patients who are failing post-operatively.

"Nothing makes you feel older faster than a bad back."
– Rickard Robert, *Men's Health*

Dr. Hubert Rosomoff is Medical Director and Renee Steele-Rosomoff is Program Director of the University of Miami School of Medicine Comprehensive Pain Center.

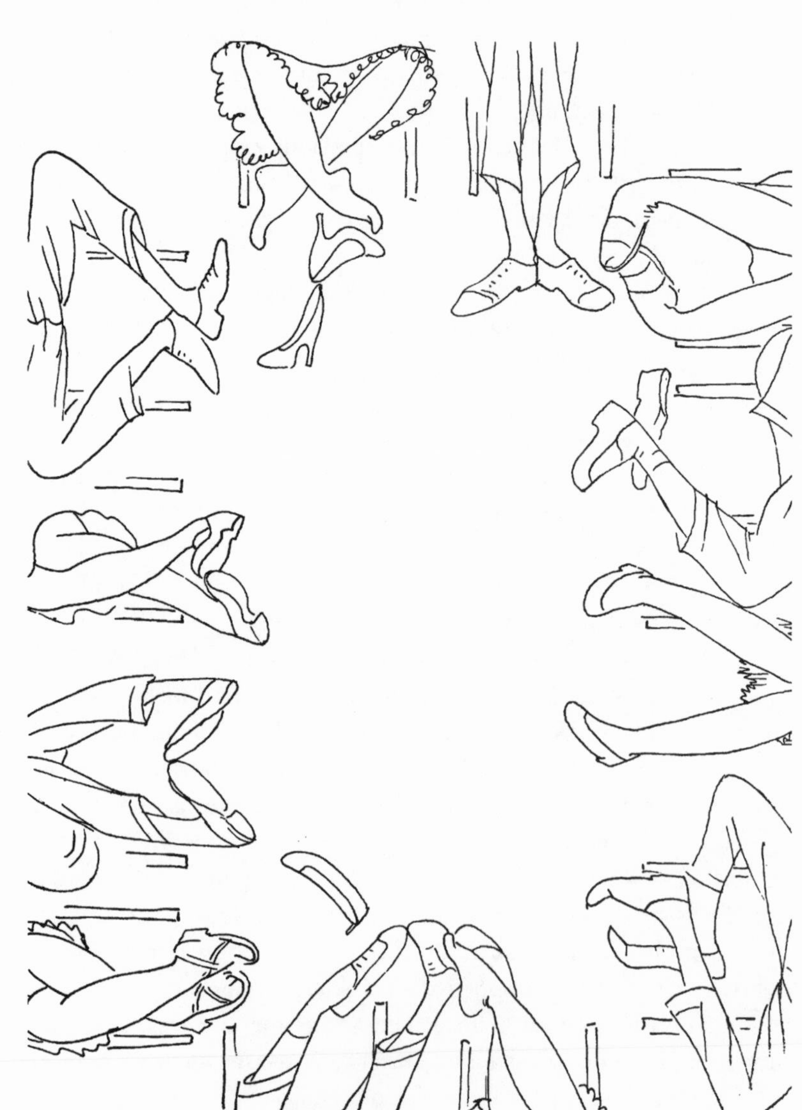

DRUG THERAPY

There are several kinds of drugs used to control low back pain. Some are mild and some are extremely strong. Some of the most commonly prescribed painkilling drugs include analgesics (pain relievers) like acetominophen (Tylenol), Darvon and Darvocet N, and Non-Steroidal Anti-Inflammatory Drugs (NSAID) like aspirin, ibuprofen, Feldene, Naprosyn and Indomethacin (very powerful!). NSAIDs are popular because they both decrease inflammation and reduce pain. However, they are also associated with gastrointestinal problems.

While not everyone will experience the undesirable side effects of these commonly prescribed pain relievers, the possibility should be considered and discussed with a health practitioner, particularly in reference to long term use. Muscle relaxant drugs are prescribed to relax tense and spasming muscles. These include drugs such as Parafon Forte DSC, Flexeril and Elavil. Anti-anxiety drugs also have a muscle relaxant ability and are quite commonly prescribed for back pain. Among these are Vistaril, Valium and Xanax. Be careful of narcotics such as Codeine, Percodan (a strong form of codeine plus aspirin) or Dialaudid (extremely strong narcotic). These are addictive drugs that should not be taken for a long time, or with alcohol, or while operating moving vehicles. (See What Works section for survey results on drug therapy.)

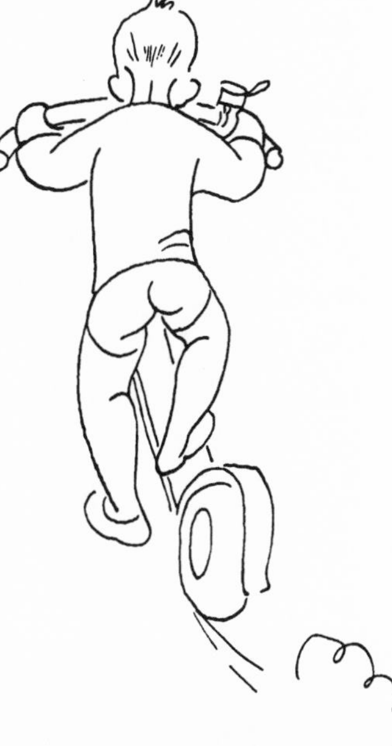

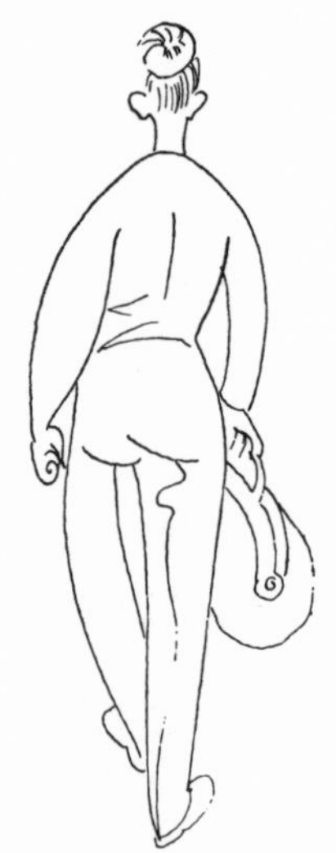

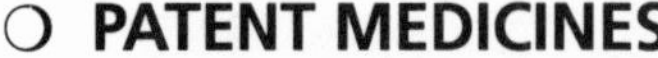

PATENT MEDICINES

Over-the-counter patent medicines abound on the market today. Commercials for Doan's rub, Ben-Gay and Heet deep heating action for sore muscles and back pain are part of our cultural experience of TV. These medicines are for the common muscle strain or sore aching muscles that can't be avoided on the job. Their roots go back to the mustard plasters of home remedies. All are applied topically (on top of the body, on the skin) and are known as external analgesics.

The effect of external analgesics are either topical analgesic, topical anesthetic, topical antipyretic (fever reducing agent) or counterirritant. Topical analgesic, anesthetic, and antipruritic agents depress skin sensory receptors for pain, itching, and burning and act directly to diminish or wipe out these symptoms on the skin due to burns, cuts, abrasions, insect bites, and other problems on the skin.

For the purposes of treating backache, the most relevant of these are the counter-irritants. In low concentrations, counter-irritants depress the skin receptors similar to the other 3 groups, but also activate and produce a mild, local, inflammatory reaction that crowds out pain messages from nearby muscles or joints. They also create heat by increasing blood flow. For this reason, these preparations should not be used with a heating pad. It may be that the real benefit from these medicines lies in the heat or massage that goes with their application allowing a respite from the hectic day, blood flowing through the muscles from the stimulation of the nerves, or just a pleasant distraction from the pain.

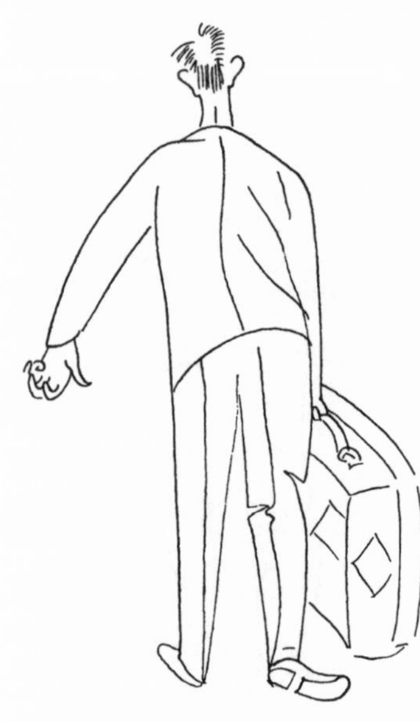

Check with your pharmacist before deciding on which patent medicine is best for you. If you have had pain for more than 3 days it could indicate a more serious problem and you should see a physician. If your pain is severe but difficult to locate, it could be referred pain indicating a problem with a different organ. If your joint is red, swollen or painful when touched, then using these medicines could delay a proper diagnosis.

These medicines work best for only minor, mild pain brought on by physical overexertion due to unaccustomed exercise or strain.

Where pain can be determined to be in one area, and you know this is not severe these medicines might be for you. If you are diagnosed by your doctor as having arthritis (something one should never determine for oneself), you might ask your doctor if these medicines might help you, in addition to your usual course of treatment.

A short list of active ingredients might take the mystique out of these medicines:

- *Allyl Isothiocyanate - volatile oil of mustard. Derived from the powdered seeds of black mustard plant and other species of mustard and can be prepard synthetically.*
- *Stronger Ammonia Water - often found diluted in liniments. Stronger ammonia water makes up smelling salts.*
- *Chloral Hydrate - a synthetically prepared agent that was used as a sedative and hypnotic before the introduction of barbitutates and other sedatives.*
- *Eucalyptus Oil - naturally occuring oil with its familiar odor. Widely used in cough lozenges.*
- *Methyl Salicylate - occurs naturally as wintergreen oil or sweet birch oil, or can be prepared synthetically.*
- *Turpentine Oil - for medicinal purposes it must be of higher quality than commercial tupentine. It is manufactured by the steam distillation of turpentine oleoresin collected from different pine trees.*
- *Menthol - extracted from peppermint oil or prepared synthetically. It is commonly used to flavor candy, chewing gum and cigarettes and as an inhalant ingredient in nasal congestion preparations.*
- *Camphor - naturally occuring in camphor trees, most is synthetically prepared.*
- *Capsicum Preparations - derived from cayenne pepper, producing a feeling of warmth.*
- *Family of Salicylates - found in aspirin, originally found in salicin (a bitter white drug found in the bark and leaves of several willows and poplars and used in medicine like salicylic acid (used in the treatment of rheumatism).*

Often two or more of these ingredients are combined to form a stronger, more active medicine. They are commonly found as liniments, gels, ointments or lotions. Make sure you read the label and follow the instructions carefully. Most recommend that they are for topical use only, avoid contact with the eyes, if pain becomes severe or lasts longer than one week see your doctor, do not use on small children under 2 years of age. Since they are counterirritants do not bandage or apply to open wounds.

"Every extra pound puts seven to 10 pounds more compression on your spine."
— Cheryl Tevis, *Successful Farming*

§ *Take breaks every 20-30 minutes when driving. A four hour drive with the best back cushion can leave you stiff and sore.*

The following is a list of common, over-the-counter medications which employ these counter-irritants:

Absorbent Rub
Absorbine Arthritic
Absorbine Jr.
Act-On Rub
Anabalm
Analgesic Balm
Aspercreme
Bamalg
Baumodyne
Ben-Gay
Ben-Gay Original
Braska
Counterpain rub
Dencorub
Doan's Rub
Emul-O-Balm
Heet
Icy Hot
Infra-Rub
Mentholatum
Minit Rub
Mobisyl
Musteroleal
Omega Oil
Sloan's
Soltice Quick Rub
Stimurub
Surin
Tiger Balm
Yage's Liniment
Zemo Liquid Regular and Extra Strength
Zemo Ointment

The above list extracted from Nancy C. Lublanezki and Robert W. Cleary, Handbook of Nonprescriptive Drugs, 8th Edition, Washington, DC: American Pharmaceutical Association, The National Professional Society of Pharmacists.

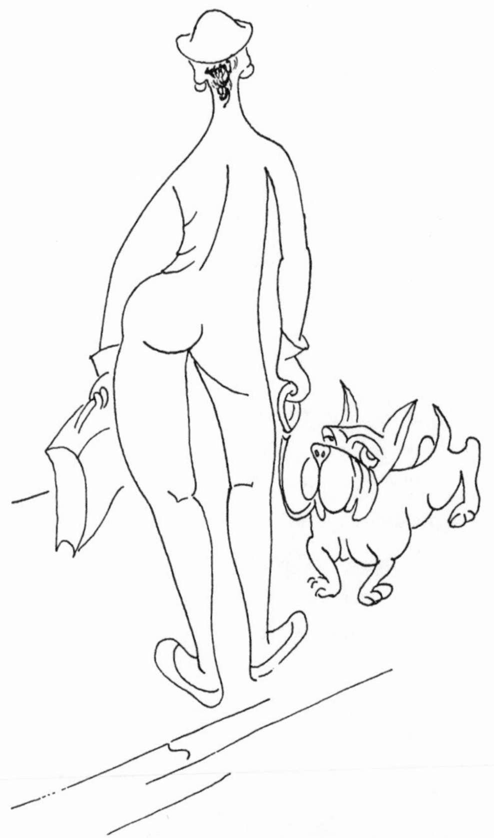

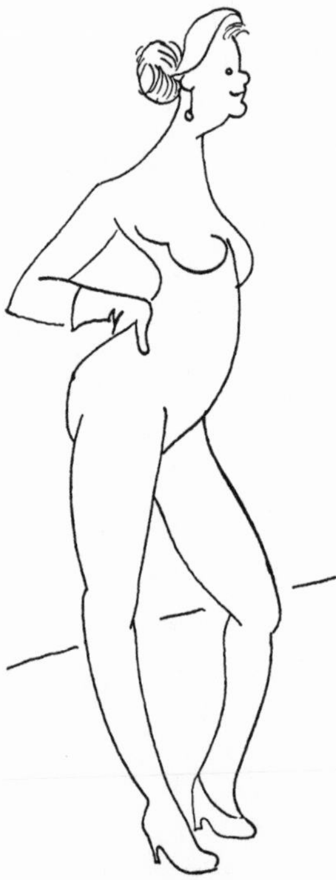

YOGA: THE WAY BACK TO HEALTH

Adapted from Back Care Basics: A Doctor's Gentle Yoga Program for Back and Neck Pain Relief *by Mary Pullig Schatz, M.D.*

WHAT IS YOGA?

Because yoga has its roots in the Hindu culture of India, there is a popular misconception that yoga is a religion. Just as practice of the Japanese martial arts of karate and aikido does not require becoming a Buddhist, the practice of yoga does not require that you adopt Hinduism. Rather, yoga is nonsectarian, promoting health and harmonious living.

Hatha yoga hands down to modern culture the art of healing the physical body through the use of a highly sophisticated array of postures, movements, and breathing techniques. The exercises take each joint in the body through its full range of motion, strengthening, stretching, and balancing each part. When practiced regularly, the yoga poses and breathing techniques promote physical and mental health.

Yoga differs from other types of rehabilitative exercise in that it engages the whole person. The yoga-based relaxation techniques and stretching and strengthening exercises in my program are effective because the mind is focused in a meditative way on your movements, skin and muscle sensations, and relaxed breathing. Mind and body work together, creating a physiological and psychological environment that optimizes the potential for healing.

One of the greatest benefits of the yoga approach is that it helps combat the negative effects of pain, disability, and stress on your mind and body. Approaching these rehabilitation exercises in a self-exploratory way helps you learn about the sources of pain in your body and their connection to your feelings, emotions, experiences, and expectations. The yoga approach to exercise provides powerful skills for coping with the ups and downs of daily life.

YOGA CLASSES AND YOGA TEACHERS

For the early stages of back rehabilitation, working with Back Care Basics on your own or privately with a trained yoga teacher is probably safest, as people tend to overdo when first starting a class. If possible, work with a yoga teacher experienced in using yoga for the rehabilitation of back injuries. After working privately for some time with this teacher, you may want to join a class for beginners. (See Resources at the end of this chapter.)

Choose a yoga teacher with care. Before participating, observe a class. Is the class small enough that everyone can move comfortable and get individual attention? Does the teacher observe each student in each pose? Does the teacher make individualized adjustments and corrections? Are the poses modified for the limitations and special needs of students? Do you like the way the teacher presents the material and leads the class? Does it look fun and enjoyable?

"Ninety-five percent of the time, you are to blame for your back problems because you don't take the time to exercise and stretch and keep your back in good condition."
– Richard M. Grossman, *Washington Post Health*

To participate safely in a class, you need a teacher who can modify poses for your requirements. It helps if the teacher has had experience with students with back challenges. Ask!

A yoga teaching certificate does not necessarily mean the teacher is qualified. Some certificates are given for attending yoga courses of only a few weeks, and many teachers receive little or no training in assessing flexibility, evaluating alignment, or adjusting poses so everyone can perform them safely. In contrast, an Iyengar-style yoga teacher's training usually includes intensive study of anatomy, physiology, yoga philosophy, and modification of poses to meet individual needs.

RELAXATION AND EXERCISE

The Relaxation Response

Although most people feel that their leisure activities are relaxing, therapeutic relaxation means practicing a set of skills that create a specific physiological response. This response is not difficult to learn, but most Westerners have to be taught it, because it is not part of our cultural heritage.

The common denominator of all inducers of the relaxation response is an internal focus. Every time the mind wanders (and it will), bring your attention gently back to the focus point. Directing attention internally is the physiological opposite of directing attention to the outside world looking for danger. When attention is directed inward, your body receives messages that you are safe and secure and that it is appropriate to relax. So muscles relax, blood pressure drops, nerves are calmed, anxiety is decreased, immunity is heightened, and healing is enhanced.

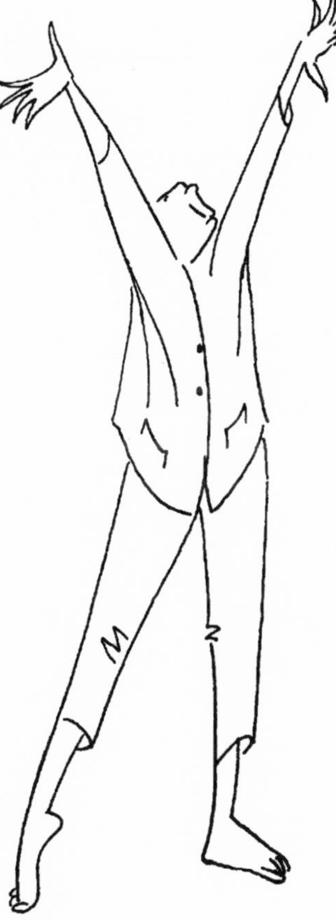

The Relaxation Breath

A number of techniques can be used to create the relaxation response. My favorite is the Relaxation Breath taught by my yoga teacher, B.K.S. Iyengar. (Others include mechanical biofeedback, progressive muscular relaxation, guided imagery, Transcendental Meditation, and other types of meditation.)

The following Relaxation Breath is elegantly simple, yet quickly and effectively produces deep relaxation. It can be practiced either sitting or lying down.

- *Step 1: Inhale naturally through your nose.*
- *Step 2: Exhale naturally through your nose.*
- *Step 3: Pause while counting to yourself, one thousand one, one thousand two.*
- *Step 4: Repeat steps 1, 2, and 3. Continue breathing in this manner for several minutes.*

You may notice a spontaneous, unforced continuation of the exhalation during step 3. This additional release of breath completes a true normal exhalation.

If possible, breathe through your nose, but, of course, if your nose is congested, you must breathe through your mouth.

Do not try to inhale deeply, exhale deeply, or breathe slowly. If you feel the urge to inhale more deeply, follow this urge and then return to normal breathing.

Whenever possible, keep your eyes closed and looking down, as if they were looking at your lower eyelids. Notice how the eyes tend to look up with each inhalation. Resist this tendency. Notice the effect of your eye position on your awareness, calmness, and ability to relax. (If contact lenses make it uncomfortable to look down, look straight ahead; just don't allow your eyes to look up.)

Most people habitually exhale incompletely, starting each inhalation without allowing the previous exhalation to come to its natural conclusion. If exhalation is allowed to conclude spontaneously and naturally, the mind does not have a chance to become agitated. When your awareness is repeatedly returned to the breathing process, the physiology of stress gives way to the relaxation response.

❍ RESTING AND RELAXING YOUR BACK

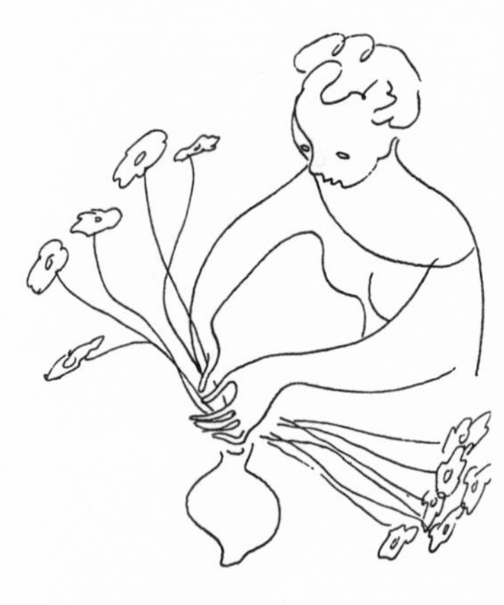

The relaxation poses described here are a good way to start doing yoga. Practice one or more of them every day, following the routines suggested. It is also a good idea to do one or two resting poses before bedtime.

Practice Relaxation poses when you feel tired or when you become aware that your posture has slipped into old habits during any activity. These poses can also help you get the kinks out after a long trip or mild trauma.

It is especially useful to practice Relaxation poses before commencing an activity that is likely to challenge your back. The postures can help you begin the potentially dangerous activity with a better alignment, so injury is less likely to occur. They can remind your muscles and bones of alignment principles, so you are more likely to use proper body mechanics as you pass through the danger zone. Afterward they can help you return to correct alignment. They may be used as a prelude and postlude to any vigorous activity, including sexual intercourse.

§ *A 2-inch piece of covered foam works very well for seat cushions if you have hardwood chairs. Make sure there is a back cushion on the one you use.*

❍ A FEW WORDS ABOUT PAIN

In performing yoga poses for lower back therapy, one should avoid creating pain or numbness in the back, buttocks, hips, legs or feet. Such pain or numbness is a warning signal that the movement being performed is damaging to the body in some way. The intensity of the position should be adjusted so that one can work without creating pain or numbness. If the warning signals persist no matter how the positions are adjusted, one should consider having another medical evaluation. In those with chronic pain who literally "hurt all the time," care should be taken to keep pain from increasing. Another warning signal for potential long-term nerve damage is muscle weakness in one leg or foot. Should this develop, medical re-evaluation is recommended.

❍ Practicing Relaxation

To practice Relaxation poses, choose a place where you will be neither too warm nor too cold. Lying on a folded quilt or blanket on the floor (rather than on a bed) is best. Be sure to use good body mechanics while getting down onto the floor and coming back up. From a standing position, firmly place one foot slightly behind the other. Using a cane or a sturdy piece of furniture as needed for support, go down on one knee, keeping your ears over your center of gravity. Then kneel on both knees. Take your buttocks back toward your heels and sit to the side of your feet. To lie down, use your arms to ease one side of your torso down to the floor; then roll onto your back. To stand, reverse this process. If the pressure of the floor on your spine, sacrum or tailbone is uncomfortable, put an extra folded towel or blanket under the tender spot.

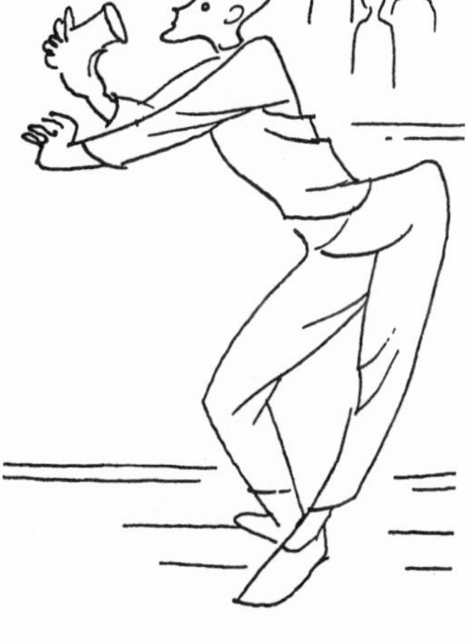

Make sure that you will not be disturbed. You will not be able to relax fully if you know that you may have to pop up to answer the phone at any moment. If you do not have an answering machine, take the phone off the hook. Let the world wait.

If the room is cool or you have a tendency to become chilled, dress warmly and have a blanket nearby. Part of the physiological response to relaxation is the opening of the blood capillaries in the skin. This creates a transient warming feeling on the skin, which is followed by chilling, as the blood loses heat to the surrounding cool air through the dilated capillaries.

❍ SUPPORTING THE HEAD AND NECK

Remember that the natural curve of the neck is convex toward the front and concave toward the back. Deep relaxation and release of muscle tension in the neck and shoulders is greatly facilitated by proper support of the cervical curve and the back of the head with carefully selected padding.

The support for the back of the neck must be firm, not soft and compressible. Rolled or folded towels and bath mats work quite well.

§ *If you get into a van or truck (something much taller) get up first, then sit down, then swing your legs in. Avoid bending and twisting as much as possible.*

§ *Carry heavy objects close to your body at your waist. Paper bags for groceries work better than plastic ones that force you to carry heavy objects at the far end of outstretched arms.*

Place a roll under your neck and a pad under your head. The roll should be low on the neck, perpendicular to the spine, with one long edge touching the tops of the shoulders.

You should feel support and comfort behind the neck, but your throat should not feel compressed (padding too thick). Nor should your throat feel overstretched (padding too thin).

❍ RELAXATION EXERCISES

Lying Down with Calves on a Chair

Props needed: chair, neck support roll, head pad, two- to four-pound weight (such as a bag of rice or dried beans).

Position and Adjustment

Lie on your back, with your calves resting on a chair seat, sofa, or other prop of an appropriate height so that your knees and your hips are bent at about ninety degrees. Place the weight on your abdomen between your waist and your pubic bone.

Make sure that your neck support roll and head pad are appropriately placed and of the proper thickness to comfortably support your spine. You may wish to place a cloth over your eyes.

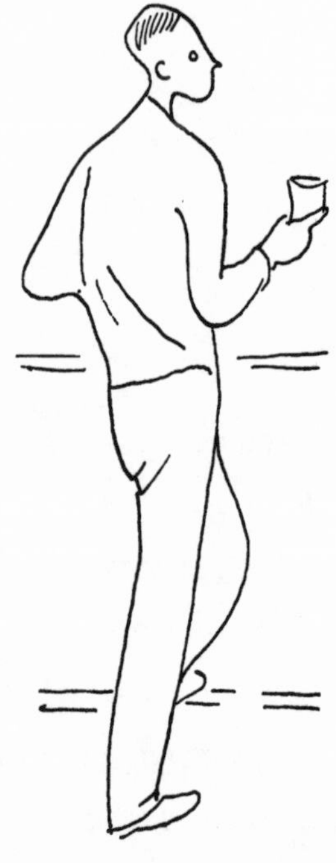

Slide your hands behind your waist and then down under your buttocks toward your legs. This will release any tension in the lumbar area by readjusting the buttock skin and flesh. Then roll your shoulders back and under, so that your arms rest comfortably with the palms facing up.

Rest here for one to five minutes. Then roll onto your side and rest there for thirty to sixty seconds before using your arms to push yourself to a seated position. Move quietly to the next pose.

Breathing and Imagery

Use the Relaxation Breath, pausing at the end of each exhalation. Keep your eyes closed and looking down, as if they were looking at your lower eyelids. Visualize your spine's normal curves being supported by the props and the floor.

Rationale

This supported Relaxation pose is especially effective for resting the lower back and shoulders. The weight on the abdomen creates a pleasant feeling of release and relaxation in the muscles and nerves of the spine.

Notes:

- *This is a good pose for those with spondylolysis or spondylolisthesis.*
- *Do not use the weight on your abdomen if you are pregnant.*
- *Do not practice this pose during the second half of pregnancy.*

Elbows on the Table

Props Needed: chair, table

Position and Adjustment

Sit in a straight chair on a nonslip surface in front of a table, so that you can comfortably lean forward onto the table. Rest your head and folded arms on the table. Avoid letting your lower back overarch. Soften your front lower ribs back into your body to slightly flatten the lumbar curve and stretch the paraspinal muscles (the muscles on either side of the spine). Hold this position for twenty to thirty seconds, breathing normally. Release and repeat several times, alternating the crossed position of the arms. (If you begin with the left forearm on top, place the right forearm on top the next time and so on.) Always return to the erect sitting position slowly, breathing deeply, to avoid dizziness.

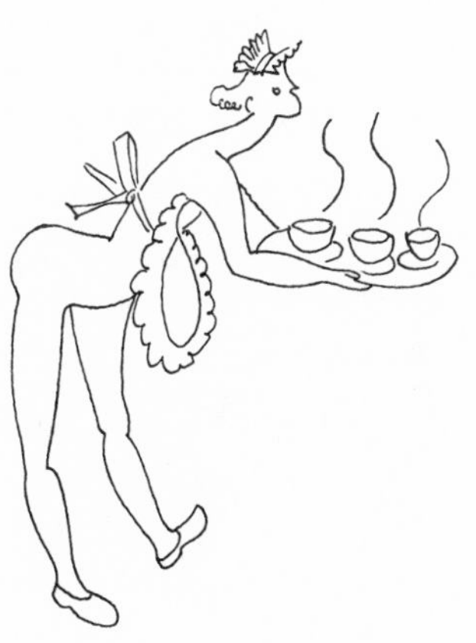

Breathing and Imagery

With each breath, allow your lower back to lengthen and release. Use the Relaxation Breath, breathing normally and pausing at the end of each exhalation for several seconds.

Rationale

This supported position allows the spinal muscles to release and lengthen so that the vertabrae can separate and allow the discs to expand. Resting the forehead in this way encourages the relaxation response by relieving the neck and shoulder muscles of their burden.

Notes:

- *If you have a flat lumbar curve, allow your lower back to arch slightly toward a more normal curve.*
- *This pose is not suitable for those with spondylolysis or spondylolisthesis.*
- *This is a great back rester for those in late pregnancy.*

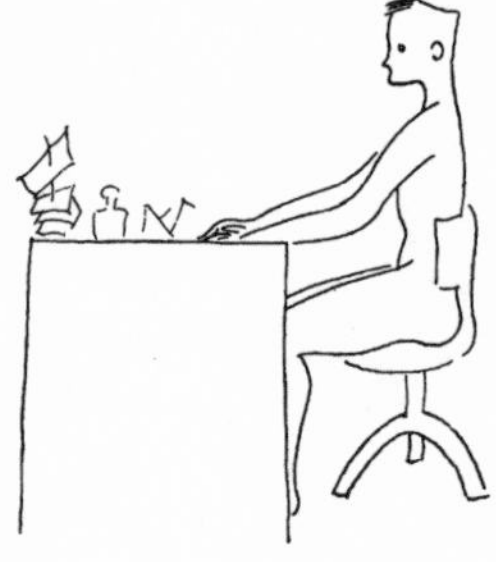

Side-Lying Relaxation

Props needed: head pad, neck support roll, two blankets

Position and Adjustment

Lie on your side, with the lower leg straight and the upper leg bent. Arrange the head pad and neck support roll. The head pad should be thick enough to fill the space between the floor, the side of your head and neck, and the top of your shoulder. (Note: This will be thicker than the support needed for the head and neck when lying on your back.) Place your upper knee and upper arm on the folded blankets. Elongate the sides of your body by stretching each hip in turn away from your lower ribs.

Breathing and Imagery

Use the Relaxation Breath. Continue to breathe your spine long with each inhalation and exhalation. Keep your eyes closed, looking down at your lower eyelids.

Stay here for two to ten minutes or as long as you are comfortable. Keep a blanket handy in case you get chilled. Return to sitting slowly to avoid dizziness.

Rationale

This is a resting pose for those who are uncomfortable lying on their backs. It is also a great sleeping position.

Note:

◇ *This is the best resting pose for the latter half of pregnancy. A pillow can be placed under the belly for additional support and comfort.*

❍ CONCLUSION

In conclusion, I would like to stress the need for an accurate medical diagnosis before proceeding with any sort of therapy for back pain. Conventional medicine does have a poor track record in the therapy of posture-related back pain, but it excels in establishing a diagnosis. If the final opinion shows that you have chronic lumbar strain or trauma, begin this yoga program.

§ *Put all materials to be typed from up on a copy holder.*

Unfortunately, there is no instant and permanent cure for back problems. By providing us with tools for observing our posture, physical as well as emotional and spiritual, yoga helps us to move in the direction of balance. Cease despising your back as your torturer and learn to accept it as your teacher. This teacher will remind you of the need to be attentive to your posture and to the conditions of life that cause you stress. Your teacher will help you monitor your progress in handling your internal as well as your external world. Give up the mantra "I have a bad back." As you practice, let your new mantra be "My back is getting healthier."

§ *Avoid lifting. Use handcarts, dollies or other devices to aid in moving and lifting materials. Handcarts and hoists are real bargains, especially compared to hospital fees.*

About the Author:

Mary Pullig Schatz, M.D., is a pathologist and certified Iyengar-style yoga teacher. She practices medicine and yoga in Nashville, Tennessee where she is Medical Staff President at Centennial Medical Center. She is a regular contributor to the "Exercise Adviser" column for The Physician and Sportsmedicine and is the author of *Back Care Basics: A Doctor's Gentle Yoga Program for Back and Neck Pain Relief* (Rodmell Press, 1992). Dr. Schatz teaches Back and Neck Care Basics Seminars℠ throughout the United States.

❍ RESOURCES

- *Back Care Basics: A Doctor's Gentle Yoga Program for Back and neck Pain Relief,* by Mary Pullig Schatz, M.D., is available from Rodmell Press, 2550 Shattuck Ave., #18-L, Berkeley, CA, 94704; 510-841-3123. $19.95, plus $3.00 shipping. (Calif. residents add 8¼% sales tax.)
- To find a yoga teacher in your area, consult the "International Yoga Teachers Directory" published annually in the July/August issue of *Yoga Journal: The Magazine for Health and Conscious Living,* 2054 University Ave., Berkeley, CA 94704; 800-359-YOGA. $5.00.
- Correspondence to Dr. Schatz can be addressed to Rodmell Press.

SEX AND BACK PAIN

Perhaps no single human activity is more important, from an emotional viewpoint, as sex. Unfortunately, sexual activity is one of the first activities to be forgone during an episode of back pain. Although acute back pain may temporarily preclude sex, there is no doubt that orgasm in itself is an excellent muscle relaxant and nature's own stress reliever. All too often people who have episodes of back pain can be apprehensive about sex, fearing more pain. Their partner may be afraid to go near for fear of making it worse. Back pain becomes the excuse not to have sex.

It is important to remember that even during an episode of extreme spasm, you can be physically close and cuddle. There are emotional and psychological benefits that both partners receive from sharing physical intimacy. The suggestions that follow are for heterosexual intercourse, since that presents the most specific physical limitations. Also bear in mind that non-coital forms of sex such as masturbation, mutual masturbation and oral sex can all be explored and may add a new dimension to your relationship.

"The best defense against future back problems is a good offense: Keep your back and stomach muscles strong."
— *Changing Times*

The first rule of good sex, a good relationship, and working through pain, is to have open, clear and honest communication. Don't be afraid, even if you're in pain, to let your partner know what your needs are. Conversely, the loving partner should understand the inherent benefits of both people feeling good. Every attempt should be made to reach out to one another. Within the nervous system, only touch has priority over pain.

As long as it doesn't hurt, it's fine. Let your pain be your guide. Worries over performance standards need to be discussed. Now is not the time for vigorous displays of power and strength. Contortionist moves are out.

§ *Make beds thoroughly on one side (tuck in sheets, blanket(s)), then move to the other side. Make sure you are on one knee, and not bending over!!! Better yet, get someone else to make them. Get help changing sheets.*

Time and patience are critical factors. Pick a time of day when you are least likely to be in pain. Start out with a relaxed setting. Put on music you like and do what it takes to put you in the mood. If your bed is associated with too much pain, try a firm bed in another room, or make a comfortable setting on the floor.

It is recommended that patients who have had back surgery, such as a fusion, should first be able to walk a mile without an increase in pain before resuming sexual activities. Pelvic motion should be kept to a minimum at first. If there is increased pain, check with your health care provider.

Be aware that if you are taking strong pain medications, they can affect your sexual arousal. You may want to decrease pain medication before sex and take it afterwards. If you have pain, don't increase your medication – change your position!

The best position is the one that causes the least pain. It may be easiest to approach lovemaking from a horizontal position, at first. The partner with back pain should be on his or her back or side. This relieves the pressure on your discs more than a standing position, and much more than in a sitting position. If your back feels better slightly arched, you may want to be on top of your horizontal partner. Your partner may need to assume a more active role. Most of all it should be enjoyable for both partners.

Both partners with back pain:

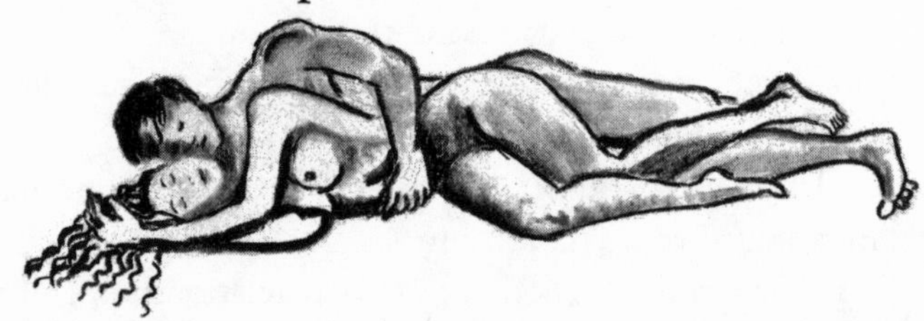

1. Side by side spoon position may work best. Both partners lie on their sides, facing the same direction. This also works very well if only one partner is in pain. (The person behind should be careful of the partner's back.)
2. The woman gets on her knees and rests her forearms on a chair. The man must stay upright on his knees that are to the inside of hers.

For the one partner with back pain:

The partner with back pain lays on his/her back. A pillow is under the head, a small towel roll under the lower back and the knees bent and supported by firmer pillows. Partners face one another. This top partner will also have to assume the active role of pelvic thrusts.

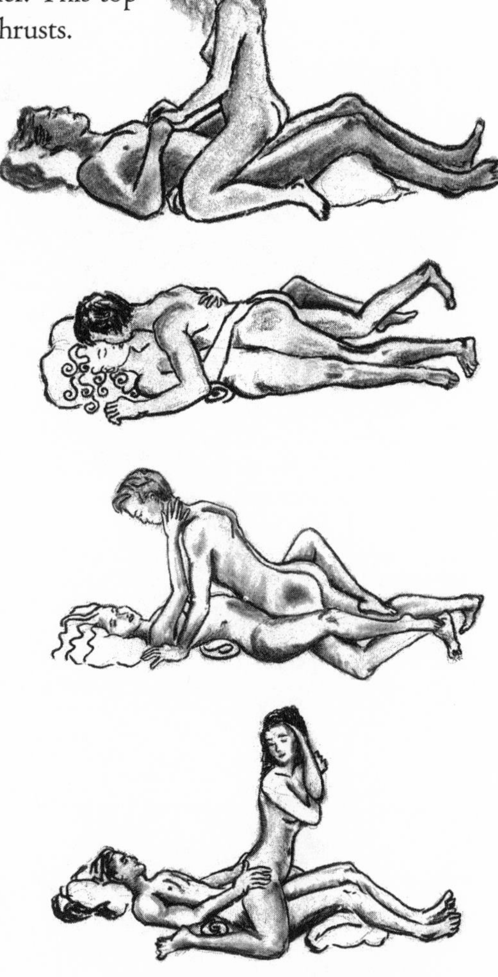

1. The woman on top takes the weight on her knees, shins and feet. Her legs are straddled on either side of his.
2. The male on top either has to keep his arms straight or take some of their weight off by resting his forearms on the bed in a more horizontal position.
3. Or, he can rest on his knees and shins with her legs over his thighs.
4. The partner with back pain lays on his/her back supported with pillows, towel roll and cushion. This time, the top partner faces away from the bottom partner, using their knees to take some of their weight off the bottom partner.

For the man with back pain only:

5. The woman gets on all fours, but drops her elbows to the bed resting on her forearms. The man then gets behind her, on his knees (with his knees to the inside of hers). Keeping his back slightly rounded, leans over her and supports his weight with straight arms on either side of her, his hands resting on the bed. This position is not recommended for the woman with back pain.

6. The man with back pain may want to try getting on his knees on the floor at the edge of the bed. The woman lays back on the edge of a low bed (her legs over the edge of the bed).

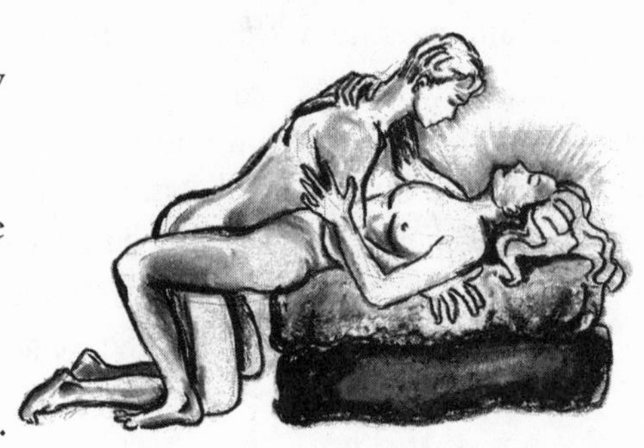

For women with back pain:

7. The partner sits in a chair, and the woman sits on his lap straddling him, face to face.

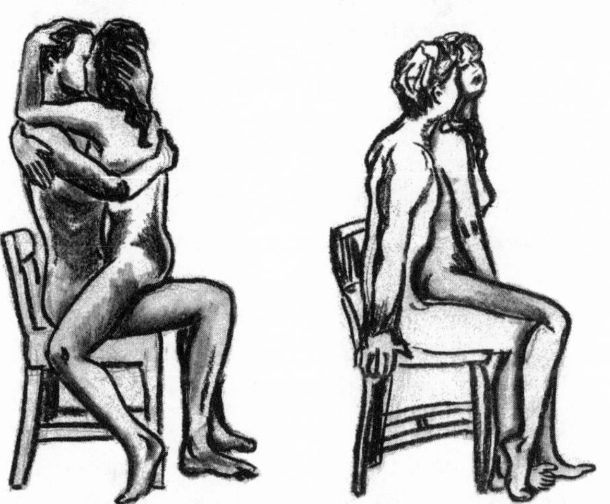

8. The partner sits down, and the woman sits on top both facing the same direction.

These positions may cause discomfort to the seated partner, especially if you both are thin.

Certainly this is not meant as a sex therapy guide or the last word on sexual positions. These are just ideas for both partners to keep in mind, and an opportunity to try experimenting to find what works for both of you. *Enjoy!*

YOUR BACK AND THE ZODIAC

Astrology by Dierdre

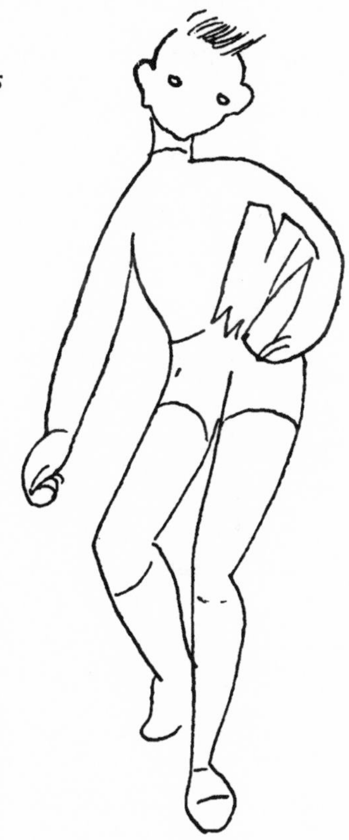

The following is a thumbnail sketch of how your sun sign and its attendent elements and modes may affect your back.

ARIES (Cardinal Fire): Aries rules the head and all born under this sign need to be careful of blows to the head. Aries can have problems related to impulsiveness and overexertion, which leads to a general tendency to be accident prone.

TAURUS (Fixed Earth): Taurus governs the neck and creates a tendency to be stubborn and literally "stiff necked." Taurans who don't direct their considerable energies in a positive way can be rigid, leading to problems with flexibility. Whiplash is a classic Taurus injury.

GEMINI (Mutable Air): Gemini rules the shoulders and arms. With their dual natures, Geminis can become unbalanced. Their natures tend toward the intellectual which can result in a loss of contact with physical reality. Beware of carrying unbalanced loads and try to maintain a strong center.

CANCER (Cardinal Water): Cancer dominates the chest, breast and stomach. Obviously, there is a tendency to top heaviness here. To avoid lower back problems, do keep those abdominal muscles in shape!

LEO (Fixed Fire): Leo controls the upper back and heart. Beware of overdoing it out of pride. Slumping, lifting improperly or lifting too much weight all pose particular threats.

VIRGO (Mutable Earth): Virgo rules digestion and intestines. A health conscious sign, Virgos have good self-discipline which, coupled with a regular exercise program, should keep them

§ *Simplify your life. If you can have groceries delivered, hire household help, or have store items sent to your house, you are way ahead of the game. Any time you can save energy, and wear and tear on your back, do it; you will have the energy to enjoy your life more fully and will improve the quality of your life.*

out of back trouble. However, a critical and anxious nature can exacerbate stiffness and problems with body alignment.

LIBRA (Cardinal Air): Libra controls the lower back and, as this sign is symbolized by scales, maintaining proper balance and posture are critical.

SCORPIO (Fixed Water): Scorpio rules the pelvis and its natives must be conscious of pelvic position, *i.e.* not standing swaybacked or balancing on one leg. Pregnant Scorpios need to be extra conscious of their posture.

SAGITTARIUS (Mutable Fire): Sagittarius dominates the hips and thighs. Sagittarian compulsiveness can lead to clumsiness and careless accidents. Beware of falls to the hip and a general tendency to get carried away by the moment.

CAPRICORN (Cardinal Earth): Capricorn controls the knees. Natives of this sign must be extra careful in choosing an exercise or sport which is easy on the knees and wear proper foot gear to minimize shock. Remember when knee injury exists, a back problem can soon follow!

AQUARIUS (Fixed Air): Aquarius governs calves and ankles which need to be strengthened and supported. Don't neglect the upper body in tending to build up the legs. Aquarians' head-in-the-clouds nature can lead to problems with lateral movement. Have your legs measured for possible inconsistencies in length.

PISCES (Mutable Water): Pisces governs the feet. Beware of tripping and use good foot support. Natives of this sign can have real trouble being grounded. They need to be aware of where they place their feet to avoid accidents and need to emphasize the physical more than is their nature to do so.

❍ THE ELEMENTS

SIGNS

FIRE with their warmth, enthusiasm and impulsiveness can speed their recovery on the mental side by maintaining a positive mental attitude. Physically, the element of warmth in heating pads, saunas, and the sun can encourage healing. They do need to guard against impatience and impulsiveness, not trying to push themselves into activities before they are fully healed.

EARTH with its intensely physically oriented nature is more in touch with the physical self than the other elements. On the negative side, illness can lead to inertia and despondency. Focusing on the earth by walking when able, gardening, sitting up against a tree, and mud packs may all prove therapeutic. Listening to the body's messages and following them also speeds healing in earth signs.

AIR signs, with their strong mental orientation can interfere with their own healing through nervous tension, depression and worry. Relaxation techniques, yoga, and biofeedback can help to reduce stress and use the mind to aid rather than hinder healing. Movement therapy, dance, tai chi and forms of suspension could also help.

WATER being a highly emotional element needs to watch going off the deep end, especially when recovering from back problems. Water based back therapies will help, such as hot tubs, moist heat pads and swimming. For general calming, a visit to the ocean gazing at the waves coming in may help, as will sitting beside a lake or stream.

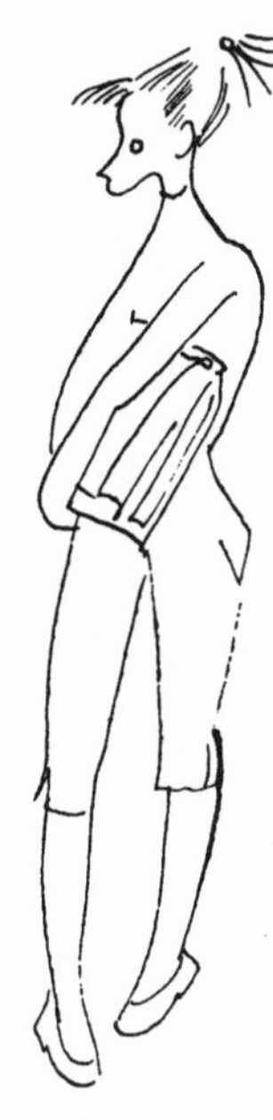

§ *It is better in the long run to make more short trips, carrying in lighter bags of groceries or supplies, then to pile them high and bust your back.*

❍ MODES

CARDINAL – Aries, Cancer, Libra, Capricorn

Tend to be energetic, go-for-it, impatient. Be sure to warm up before exercising, beware of being overambitious or doing impulsive movements (lunging, for example).

FIXED – Taurus, Leo, Scorpio, Aquarius

Be sure to develop an exercise program, as fixed signs can tend to be creatures of habit and sink into inertia. But beware of overtraining or overexercising and not knowing when to quit even a good thing.

MUTABLE – Gemini, Virgo, Sagittarius, Pisces

Tend to be easily bored, to crave change, and can have trouble sticking to things like back exercises and treatment programs necessary for full recovery after a back injury. Acting and moving without thinking can also slow progress and cause a relapse.

To Contact Dierdre Please write to Dierdre Frank, 5862 Robin Hood Drive, El Sobrante, CA 94803

BACK PAIN IN THE EMERGENCY ROOM

By David I. Greenly, MD, FACEP

Emergency Department management of back pain is limited to three narrowly defined areas: fracture, infection or nerve damage. Once these three entities are "off the table," Emergency Department management encompasses pain management only.

Usually the Emergency Physician will be able to ascertain whether or not you have "broken your back" by physical examination. After a diagnosis, x-rays may or may not be ordered. The majority of patients with acute back pain sustaining no or minimal trauma do not require x-ray evaluation. Occasionally x-rays will be ordered to determine whether or not there is "bone damage."

Attendant to bone damage is the question of whether or not there is any impingement on the nerves coming out of the spinal column through the bones of the back. Assessment of nerve dysfunction can almost always be determined on some level by the physical examination. CT scans, MRI scans, *etc.*, are all tertiary examination methods and are not routinely utilized within the Emergency Department. It is the *rare acute low back pain that results in nerve damage.*

Infection in a bone or a disc space in the back has the potential to be a dangerous situation and every Emergency Physician strives to rule out infection early in the patient encounter. The hallmark of infection in all parts of the body, not just the back, is pain and tenderness. Pain is what the patient *feels* from the area; tenderness is what the clinician can *elicit* from the affected part. Blood counts, sedimentation rates, *etc.*, are some of the screening lab tests that may or may not be ordered to rule out infection. However, if it is not tender to the touch, the overwhelming odds are that it is not infected.

§ *Get out of bed by rolling onto your side at the edge of your bed. Use your arms to raise your upper body as you lower your legs. You want to use your body as a lever: as the top part of your body comes to a sitting position, swing your legs down simultaneously.*

Once fracture, infection, and nerve damage are ruled out, the Emergency Department visit is limited to pain relief. Patients presenting to Emergency Services with complaints of back pain of an acute nature have reasonable expectations to leave the Emergency Service pain-free. Our culture at the present time tends to undermedicate patients who are in pain. There are many reasons for this. One reason is the fear of litigation from patients who might fall and hurt themselves while under the influence of medication. Another is the cultural proclivity to go light on the prescribing of narcotics. In the acute setting, adequate pain relief is a must.

Adjunctive to narcotic administration, there are many other types of pain medication on the market. Many of these medications help to relieve the symptoms of low back pain. Non-steroidal anti-inflammatory drugs (NSAIDs – Motrin, Advil, *etc.*) give relief in many situations. In addition, ice packs in the early stages of back pain, and heat and massage in the later stages of back pain may provide relief.

About the Author:

Dr. David I. Greenly is Medical Director, Emergency Services at Alta Bates-Herrick Hospital in Berkeley, California.

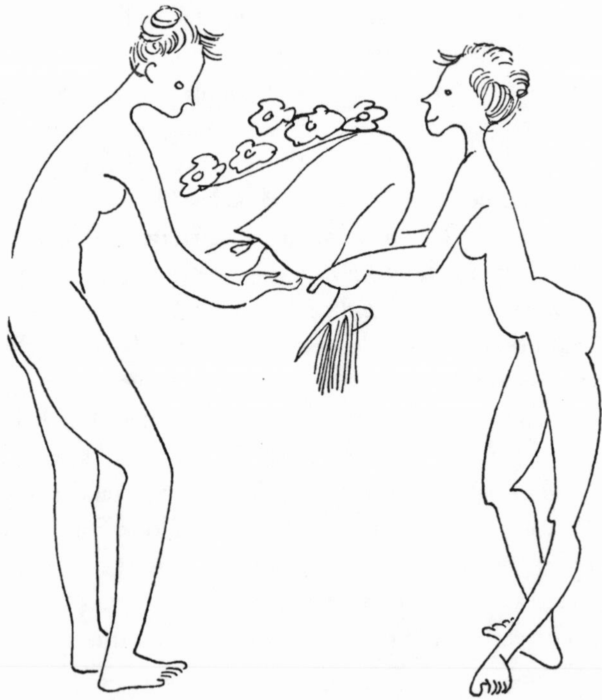

DISASTER FIRST AID

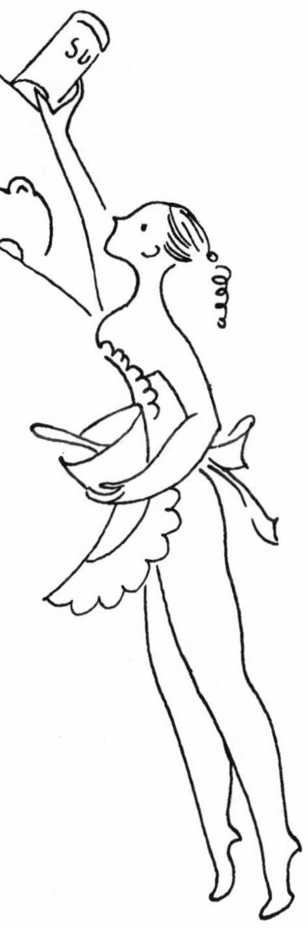

Do not move the victim unless you absolutely have to. The overriding concept is to maintain the "in line" configuration of the vertebral column – head to buttocks. If there is immediate danger, try to get the victim and yourself to a safe place (see Moving the Victim). Then check to see if there is massive bleeding (get the cleanest cloth and apply pressure directly over the wound), check to see if the victim is breathing and whether they have a pulse. Cover them lightly. Call for emergency help. Give the dispatcher all your information and let them hang up first.

❍ WATER ACCIDENTS

Always see if professional help is available, a lifeguard, off-duty lifeguard or someone trained in water rescue.

Do not attempt to rescue anyone who is in water over your head if you can't swim well and tread water for some time.

If you suspect someone has hit their head on a submerged object and is unconscious in water over your head and they are

Laying face down:

Cup their chin with one hand and the back of the skull with the other laying your forearms to your elbows, along their spine. Slowly turn them over being careful to keep your forearms parallel (don't twist them).

Once the victim is on their back:

Check to make sure they are breathing. If they aren't breathing, give mouth to mouth resuscitation, being careful to support their head and neck by cupping their head and laying your forearms along their spine. Swim to their head, and reach both your hands under the head and grasp them firmly at their underarms. Cradle their head with your forearms, elbows together, and lay back swimming them in with both of you on your backs.

Laying face up:

See once the victim is on their back above.

If your feet are touching bottom you can change back to cupping the back of their head with one hand, their chin with the other, and lay your forearms along their spine. Be careful to keep your forearms, to the elbow, parallel to each other along their spine. Do not twist this grip on their head. You can rest them on the shore as soon as their face is out of water and out of the way of waves or other dangers. Do not attempt to lift or carry them. Yell or go for help if there is no one around.

○ MOVING THE VICTIM

§ *Put on clothing that goes over your head by putting the garment over your head first, then put your arms in. Likewise, when taking off garments, take your arms out of the sleeves first, then take it off over your head.*

Don't! Unless they are in immediate danger, don't move a victim. You must always assume spinal injuries. More damage occurs from improper moving of the victim than by any other emergency aid measure. If you absolutely must move a victim because a car is on fire and about to blow up, or they are in more danger if you leave them, pull them longways by grasping them under their shoulders, or if necessary, by the feet supporting their head. Make sure you keep their body in a straight line, remembering the "in line" concept. Don't pull them sideways, or by their clothing. Don't bend, twist or shake any of their body parts.

Anyone with suspected spine, back, neck, pelvis or leg fractures or damage should be moved laying down. Splint all suspected broken or fractured parts first then move them on a backboard. Hold broken parts together while someone else moves them. It is best to wait until trained help arrives before ever moving the victim unless there is immediate danger.

LIFESTYLE AND THE WORKPLACE

One-third of each day is spent at work. For homemakers, the hours are even longer. Back problems now account for as much as one-fourth of all lost work days, and those numbers don't take the unpaid homemaker into account. No one is immune. Virtually every field of employment involves the manual tasks which are the most frequent causes of back complaints: bending, lifting and twisting. Back trouble strikes the computer operator, dry cleaning worker, homemaker and trucker with equal, and equally debilitating, swiftness.

§ *Use luggage with wheels. Use luggage dollies. It is well worth it to pay a porter to help with bags, rather than spend lots of time and money being laid up.*

Recently, the U.S. Department of Labor conducted a survey of 900 workers in blue-collar jobs who sustained back injuries associated with lifting. Included were shipping and receiving workers, stock clerks, craft worker operatives, transport operatives, and farm laborers. Jobs that included lifting humans, *i.e.,* nursing, were not included in this study.

Three fourths of the workers were between 20-40 years old. One-third were between 25-34 years old. These are workers at their peak earning years that are encountering back injuries.

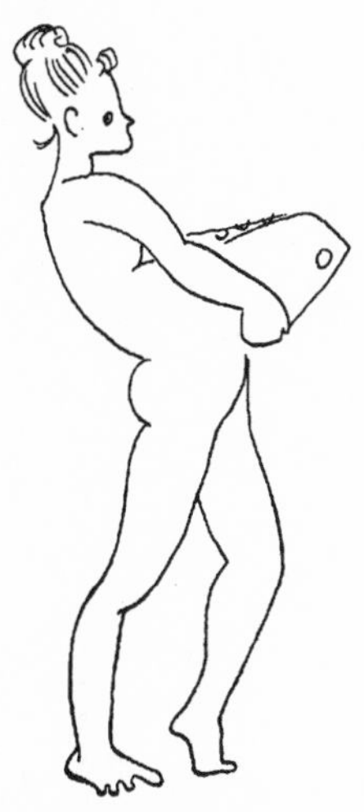

Three-fourths of the respondents stated that they were lifting at the time they injured their backs. The weight of the object was cited more often than any other factor as contributing to back injuries. Body movement was cited next as the leading cause of back injuries. Bending, twisting and turning in combinations, were most often cited as movements that caused problems. Other contributing factors were: bulkiness of the object, and lack of material handling equipment to lift and transport the objects. Two-thirds of the workers reported that they held or carried the object less than one minute.

A staggering forty-eight percent of these workers reported a history of back problems. Even more surprising was the fact that one-half of these workers had received information on how to avoid injuries while lifting through posters or written handouts, as well as through lectures, demonstrations, films or as part of the on-the-job training. The figures do not indicate how many of those with previous back trouble who received information on correct lifting procedures still injured themselves. Seventy percent of all respondents, though, had not followed any exercise program to minimize injuries to the back.

"Annual cost of back pain to U.S. economy is $60 billion. . . Percentage of U.S. population that will suffer back pain in their lives is 85 percent. . . Back pain's ranking as a cause of worker's compensation claims is no.1."
– Brendan Boyd, *San Francisco Chronicle*

Muscle strain or sprain was the diagnosis in a vast majority of the back injuries. Fourteen days was the average time lost from work. Upon return to work, more than two-fifths of the workers who had returned to work were given light duties.

This study suggests that a large portion of the population who perform manually-oriented jobs that have received information on taking care of their backs are still injuring themselves and are still not following any regular exercise or fitness program. As a result, they are losing time from work and even needing to change jobs.

Here are some simple suggestions to prevent injury on the job, whatever kind of work you do. As important, though, if you have a history of back trouble, is what you do off the job to prepare your back for your on-the-job tasks:

When you LIFT:

- *get close to the object*
- *bend your knees and hips (get down on one knee if you have to)*
- *tighten your abdominal muscles when you lift – since you have no ribs in your lower back, your abdominal muscles are your only support*
- *avoid twisting when you lift – remember to keep your shoulders square with your hips*
- *lift with your legs, not your back*

When you TWIST (fixing pipes, opening valves, etc):

- *get to an even level with the object – don't bend over it*
- *use your legs and arms, not your back*
- *keep your spine in line*

When you BEND:

- ◇ *bend your knees or get down on one knee*
- ◇ *move forward from the hips*

When you REACH:

- ◇ *reach to the right with your right hand, to the left with your left hand, for cleaning, mopping, retrieving objects, etc.*
- ◇ *get a step stool or ladder to reach anything above your shoulders*
- ◇ *check the weight by pushing up on one side before trying to bring something down*
- ◇ *tighten your stomach muscles and lift with your upper body strength*
- ◇ *as you bring the load down, let your legs absorb the weight*

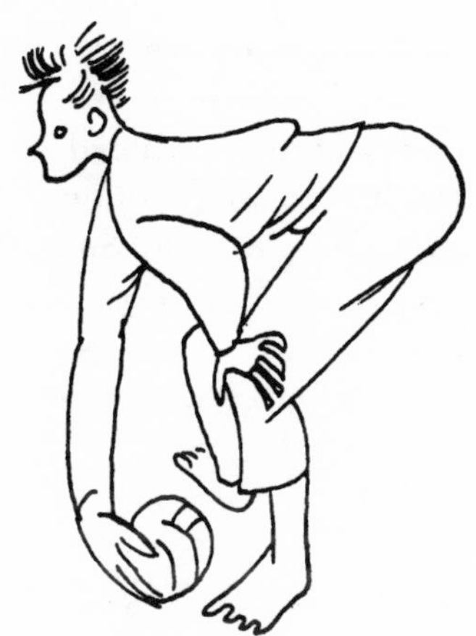

When you LOAD or STOCK:

- ◇ *keep the loads light*
- ◇ *turn your whole body to face the load and then turn to face the destination – don't twist*
- ◇ *tighten stomach muscles to lift*
- ◇ *lift with your legs and arms*

When you PUSH or PULL:

- ◇ *push instead of pull when you can*
- ◇ *keep the load close to your body – don't lean out to it or forward over it*
- ◇ *keep stomach muscles tightened*

It's only common sense to get help lifting, carrying, pushing or pulling something that seems too heavy to handle alone. No time is saved if you have to go to the doctor and someone else has to finish your job.

The above suggestions are especially important to those working in jobs like nursing, trucking, retail, maintenance and other physically taxing occupations. Office workers and students, however, are not immune to back pain either. Sitting while working, often in an uncomfortable chair, hunched over a desk or staring at a computer screen, can wreak havoc on your neck, shoulders, upper and lower back. People in sitting jobs should get up and move around at least once every hour, preferably more. And books or screens should be visible to a person sitting in an upright position. There are stretches you can do while sitting at your desk which can help to rest your back. (See the chapter on Yoga: The Way Back To Health. Another excellent reference is Donkin's *Sitting on the Job*. See our recommended

§ *Don't bend over your work. Your head is attached to your neck and shoulders and spine. If you're bending your head, you're probably rounding your shoulders as well.*

reading list.) There is an increasing amount of information on working with Video Display Terminals (VDTs). Ask your health practitioner. There is also an increasing interest in ergonomics in the workplace – fitting the furnishings to you and not the other way around.

Every job has a most efficient way to do it. It's rarely the fastest way. Take the time to consider the long term effects of your job on your body.

"Studies in Sweden found that sitting is second only to a combined bending-twisting motion for putting pressure on back muscles and ligaments."
– Joseph Alper, *Washington Post Health*

❍ LIFESTYLE AND YOUR BACK

Go easy. Reducing stress helps to lessen muscle tension which may be causing some or all of your pain. Back trouble is nature's way of warning you that you haven't learned good posture, haven't exercised (especially to keep the abdominal muscles in shape), haven't asked for help when the job is too big, or haven't slowed down your pace. And, if you haven't learned these things, then you are doomed to repeat the same mistake or pay for it dearly later. A few minutes of doing nothing, meditating, just listening to calming music, visualization (visualizing your pain as a bird that flies away, for example) or "quiet time" works as well for adults as it does to quiet down youngsters. For more information on Simple Changes you can make in your lifestyle to reduce the stress and strain on your back, send for our *free* Simple Changes information packet. (See the last page of the book.)

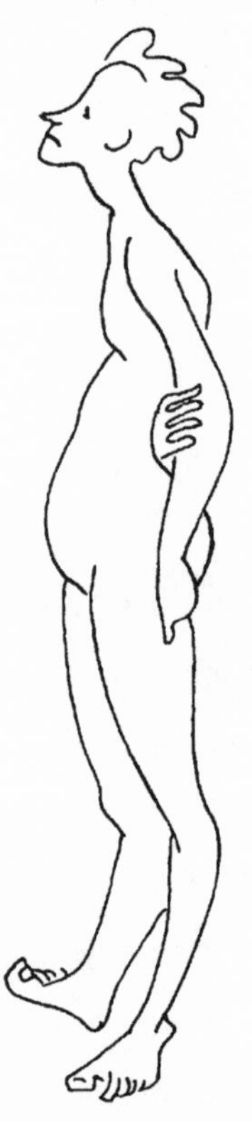

❍ POSTURE AND BODY MECHANICS

The old adage that an ounce of prevention is worth a pound of cure couldn't be more true than in reference to back pain. Posture and the position of your body is everything! Try to get to the point where you can see yourself, as if watching your life on a movie screen. Take a good look in a mirror, or catch your reflection in a store window. Are you slouched over, rushing somewhere? Use your abdominal muscles to hold in your stomach and support your lower back (there is little else supporting your lower back below your ribs). Stand up tall, think of a helium balloon being attached to the top of your head. Keep your neck long in the back, chin straight ahead. Keep your shoulders back and down. Your arms should lie relaxed at your sides. Now relax about 10% – otherwise the military pose keeps your muscles tensed and you can't hold this pose for long. The more you practice good posture the more natural it will seem.

It is usually the simple things we overlook: standing up tall, sitting up straight, both feet flat on the floor, using good body mechanics to reach something on the floor. These are some of the most important things we can learn. They affect us every day, and done incorrectly, can quickly add up to pain. It is the cumulative effects of our bad habits that most often will land us in bed with a bad back. Unfortunately, we are always looking for the fast food solution – a couple of aspirin and we're back in action. We are not taught how best to use our bodies in school or at home. Listen to your body. Unless there is some trauma or underlying disease, a physical therapist or good back school may be all you need.

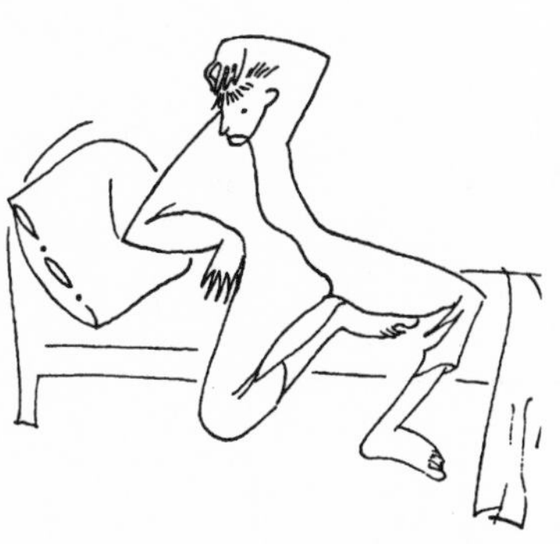

Make sure you instill in your children the benefits of an active life, good nutrition, and good posture. Teach them what you know. As early as grade school, children sit any which way in class. Taller children (most often the girls, as early as 9 or 10 years of age) are already slouching. If correct posture is taught at an early age, it will be second nature as children grow up. Part of the difficulty in changing our habits as we get older is that we've grown used to poor posture and so it seems more comfortable. If you can work through the first month or two of an awkward, uncomfortable but beneficial position, then it will seem more comfortable as time goes on. Be patient with yourself. If you have years of bad habits to break, it won't happen overnight. (See the Mensendieck section on posture.)

❍ GET UP!

Get up and move around. Today's lifestyle consists of sitting down to breakfast or rushing out the door without breakfast, sitting down on the way to work (whether we drive or take public transportation), sitting on the job, returning home (still sitting), sitting down to dinner, then "laying back" and watching TV. This sedentary lifestyle, combined with little or no exercise, poor posture and bad sleeping habits (like sleeping on your stomach) causes much of the lower back pain today. It is no wonder that reaching for the remote can cause excruciating pain.

§ *If you need to work at a desk or table, take a seat – don't lean over!*

If you sit all day long, get up every 20-30 minutes and walk around. Break up jobs and alternate body positions: after half an hour at the computer you should switch to a standing job for half an hour. If you're working at a desk, bent over, alternate with opposite movements like standing up and doing tasks that are above waist level like watering plants or dusting shelves. Change positions frequently

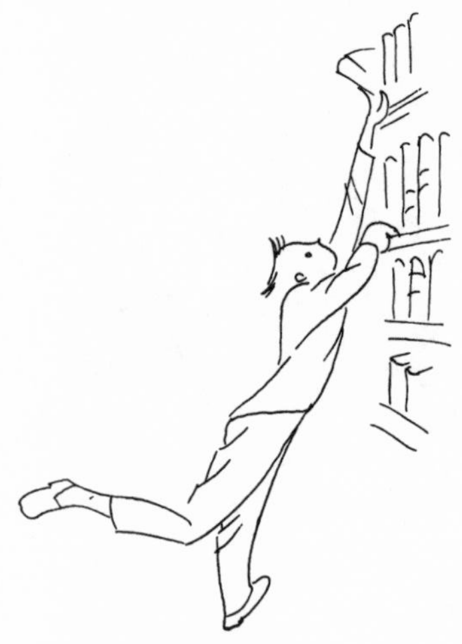

or you can become "frozen" in one position. The result is that you will feel tired, stiff and sore all over when you do get up. If you must remain seated, do some simple exercises. (See the Relaxation exercises in the yoga section.)

If you're in great pain because your back just went out, don't lay on a sagging mattress or a soft couch and wait for the pain to go away. Too much time on that sagging mattress or soft couch may be a large part of your problem. Even if you've begun to make some important changes, like making regular trips to the gym, returning home to spend the evening slumped in front of the TV may undo the good work you've done. Make sure, at the very least, that your favorite TV chair provides firm support. But better yet, find activities you enjoy that encourage movement and variation of body position.

❍ WORK SIMPLIFICATION

Besides learning to ask for help when you and your back could use it, there are some basic principles that you can apply to your home and business activities that will greatly alleviate back strain. With a little bit of planning, you can arrange your day and your work areas to avoid excess motion, and allow your back some relief from the minor stresses of everyday activities. Work simplification principles can be applied to every space you use frequently, from kitchen, to bathroom, to closet, to car. Take some time to make your life simpler.

Organize your work spaces into areas of easy reach (elbows bent and close to body) and maximum reach (each arm extended full length). Keep the articles most commonly used within easy reach, slightly less commonly used articles within maximum reach, and infrequently used articles outside of the maximum reach zone. In the kitchen, for example, store food, utensils and equipment needing water near the sink. Keep your baking ingredients and utensils together. Keep all food and utensils used first with heat in a cooking area, including canned foods, tea and coffee, pot holders, skillets. Get duplicates of items like measuring utensils which are frequently used in more than one area. Don't clutter your work space with a serving dish you use once a year.

§ *Stand tall, sit straight, and don't bend over from the waist.*

In all your work areas, keep heavy items at waist level, and use your legs to lift. Create a variety of work surfaces, including surfaces that are waist high and elbow height when standing. Having a variety of work surfaces can help you to take a rest when you need it, if not by stopping work then by switching work stations. Remember to use your right hand to reach things on your right side and your left hand to reach things on your left. Work simplification can make a huge difference by the end of a busy day. For more information, write for our free packet. (See back page.)

❍ WORKPLACE ADJUSTMENTS

§ A back cushion on your favorite chair at home. Or check out some of the new ergonomically designed furniture. You don't have to give up that rocking chair. Just pad the bottom and get a back cushion.

Many businesses have learned the value of holding back seminars in an effort to prevent on the job back injuries. Check out your company's programs. You may want to request that such a class be held for you and your co-workers. If you own the company, you may want to invest in a preventive health care class on this topic. It is much less expensive to provide preventive care than to provide long-term medical care or lose employees to the worker's compensation system and have to train new employees. Even the most sedentary workers could benefit from a back program.

Back schools often use a principle called work hardening. Back pain sufferers are trained specifically for the demands of their job or, with the cooperation of their employers, adapted to another position within their ability. Even without a back school, you can apply work simplification principles to your business environment, whether you work at a desk or in a warehouse. Think about easy and maximum reach areas and planning your day to avoid excess motion. (See Corporate Back Schools).

❍ MENTAL ATTITUDE

Pain is an enormously powerful force. It will take up all the room you allow it to in your brain so that you can't think of anything else. The more you try to find a way through it, around it, over it, the more it controls you rather than you controlling it. The more you think about it, the more you worry, the more you feel stress, the more stress creates muscle tension, the more pain you're in. It is a vicious downward spiral of pain feeding on itself.

Take control! To some extent, your pain is all in your head. You have the ability to make yourself happy or completely miserable. A positive outlook is a sure way to feel better, even if not 100% well. Complaining, and feeling miserable is the surest way to make those around you miserable as well. Try asking your friends and family to

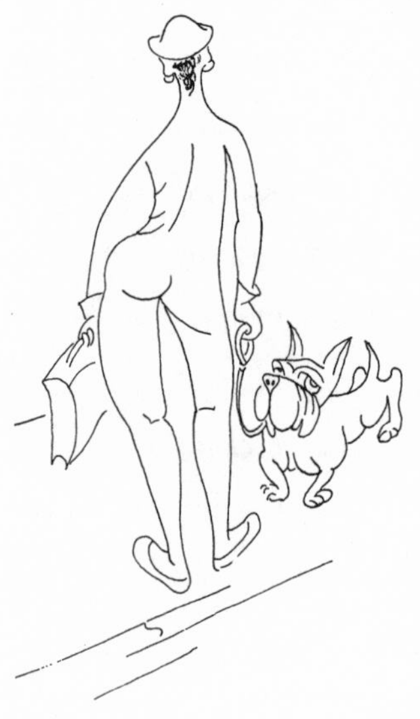

stop asking how your back is. You may have just managed to put your pain out of your head, and here you are having to think about it in order to give them an honest answer. Believe and trust that people are there for you and will lend a helping hand if you ask. You may be in pain, in bed, about to lose your job, but think of anything else. A funny video, flowers, joke books, a touching drawing from your child might help relieve the tension and subdue the pain. Breathe deeply. Relax into the pain. Breathe in, breathe out and repeat a positive phrase like "pain go away." Or imagine your pain as a bird flying away, going farther with each exhalation.

Take a look at how common sayings apply to your life: " – is on my back", " – is a pain in the neck", " – have my back against the wall", " – is spineless", " – can't stand up to anyone or anything." Do these relate to your life? Is it your job, the kids, your spouse, the neighbors? Backache with no apparent cause may be emotionally caused.

Don't allow yourself to be victimized, by others or by your own feelings of frustration and powerlessness. Take control over your situation by seeking solutions to these problems, large or small. Maybe an assertiveness training class (often taught at the local junior college) can help you take control of your life. Assertiveness training teaches you how to consider yourself before saying yes to things you don't have time for. Maybe personal, couple or family counseling will help you make some necessary changes to reduce the stress in your life. Don't be afraid to have a wonderful, pain-free life. Work to find a solution that works for you.

❍ HUMOR

Above all, don't lose your sense of humor. Laughter is the best medicine with only positive side effects. No matter how bleak it seems, you will see the light at the end of the tunnel. Hopefully it's not an oncoming train.

❍ DIET

A healthy diet is essential for your body to maintain itself and respond well to daily wear and tear. Healthy eating includes whole grains, fresh fruits and vegetables, and protein. Eat when you are hungry, and in relation to how sedentary or active your life is. There is no reason to eat like a linebacker if you're a computer programmer. Lose weight, if necessary, to take the strain off your back. Being 20 lbs overweight is equal to carrying around a 20 lb. weight. Extra weight carried in the abdomen – from a pot belly or pregnancy – causes the lower back to arch. The more weight you carry around, the more pressure is exerted on the muscles and discs of the lower back.

Try to take the time to eat three meals a day, preferably eaten without reading, watching TV or while on the move walking or driving. This will help you maintain a relatively steady blood sugar level, thus reducing stress on your body, as well enabling you to enjoy your food and better regulate the quantities you consume. If you know you're not eating right, find a vitamin supplement. This can be a complex procedure of reading, analyzing and discussing the options with a health worker, or a simple one of taking a readily available and relatively inexpensive vitamin supplement.

§ *Change uncomfortable positions frequently. If you have been kneeling, bending forward or sitting for a period of time get up and gently arch backwards.*

To take the best care of your back, make sure your diet includes:

Calcium

Calcium keeps the bones healthy, bone loss down, and can keep osteoporosis away. Two-thirds of a quart of milk, cheese, yogurt and other dairy products, green leafy vegetables (like spinach), broccoli, herring, mackerel, salmon, sardines, soybeans, tempeh, tofu, and brewer's yeast all contain calcium. Incorporate your favorites foods from this list into your daily diet. You're not fooling anyone but yourself if your daily calcium intake is the cream in your coffee and ice cream for dessert. The sugar and fat in this diet will do you more harm than any benefit you might obtain from the small amount of calcium. If this is the extent of your calcium intake, you might want to consider a calcium supplement.

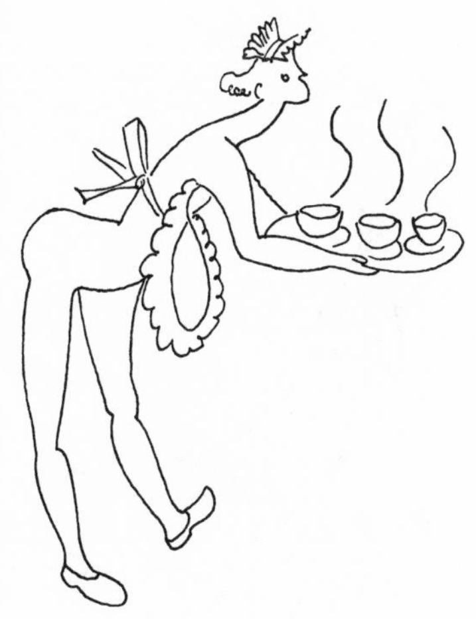

Low calcium levels can be caused by dietary and extra-dietary factors: if you eat a lot of food containing the preservative EDTA, which can prevent iron from assisting in calcium metabolism; if you're on a high protein diet; if you perspire a great deal or live in an area of high temperatures; if you live in a big city or an industrial area, or you're frequently exposed to toxins at your workplace; if you smoke, or live or work with people who smoke; or if you're regularly taking steroids. Lack of calcium could be the cause: if your muscles cramp even when you're not moving about; if your bones ache and you can't blame the weather; if you're a woman who has had minor backackes and your mother or grandmother suffered from osteoporosis in old age or had bone fractures. (For more on this subject, see *Your Personal Guide to Vitamins and Minerals,* Rodale Press)

§ *Remember, pillows are for your head; pull the pillow up off your shoulders. Soft feather pillows that can be molded to fit under your neck are wonderful.*

Water

Who really drinks 8 glasses a day? Most of us probably don't but there are good reasons why we should, especially if we have back problems. Our discs are 80% water and begin to dry up between ages 30-40. Drinking water helps to replenish discs and maintain them at optimum efficiency. Also when you drink water, toxins are removed from the body by the kidneys. As you get older, and your kidneys become less efficient, your body needs more water to keep it healthy. If drinking water is hard for you, start slowly and gradually increase your daily intake. And remember, water, not just any liquid, is what your body needs. Coffee, black tea, and alcohol are all diuretics – they cause the body to excrete fluids thus reducing body fluid levels. Drinking an iced coffee or beer on a hot day may be cool and refreshing (and tasty) but it doesn't do the work of a healthy liquid.

❍ BEDS

Whatever works for you is what's best, but if you've been waking up in pain every morning, then it may be that your bed's not working. But before you go buying a special hospital bed for back patients, try some changes in your own bedroom. Everyone's heard about the dangers of a bed that's too soft, but a bed that's too hard and doesn't conform to your body can be just as bad. It's like sleeping on the floor. A hard piece of wood under a soft mattress might be all that is needed. Futons have been touted as the new age natural solution to foam mattresses. However, futons were designed to be taken out and fluffed up each day, which requires quite a bit of time and energy since futons are heavy. If you already own a futon and it works for you, don't toss it out. If it gets too hard, you may want to try putting an equal size piece of convoluted (or egg-crate) foam over it. If softness seems to be the problem and your mattress is fine, maybe it's the box springs. Try putting your mattress on a platform bed (easily made as an upside- down bookcase).

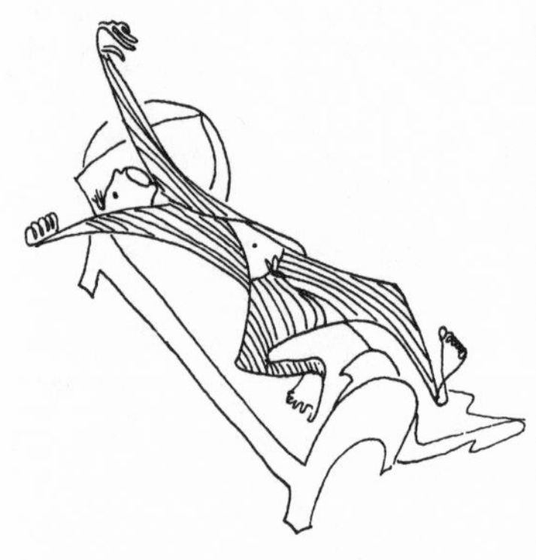

If you have difficulty getting up and down, a bed whose height comes to the back of your knees will greatly help. Getting in and out of a mattress on the floor can be difficult, and twisting to get up or lay down can be unbearable if you're in pain. However, those in lofts seem to make do with "crawling into bed". Some people swear by the floor itself – though if you're thin, your bones may ache by morning.

§ Bending over constantly to pick things up (paper, toys, clothing, etc.) will wear you out and increase back pain.

One suggestion: try a 4-5 inch hard foam with 2-inch convoluted foam on top. For appearance and convenience, this can be placed in a mattress cover. Place the foam on top of a wood platform bed. Convoluted foam, once hard to find outside of hospitals is now readily available in foam shops, hospital supply stores and by mail order (see catalog listing in resource section).

One of the greatest aids can be a simple wooden handrail built on the side of the bed. It should gradually slope up toward the headboard. This is particularly helpful to those who have just had surgery but can be a great help anytime that getting up and down or turning in bed becomes painful.

❍ EXERCISE

Exercise that strengthens the muscles of the back and abdomen is the best kind of preventive medicine for back trouble. Ask your doctor or physical therapist about low impact exercises that help to strengthen those areas where you are the weakest (whether it is the abdominal muscles, upper chest, thighs or upper arms).

It is unadviseable to start any exercise or sports program without first consulting a health care worker. Some exercises can actually increase pain. Remember, pain is a body's way of telling you that something is wrong. Before you start your exercise, think about warming up, especially first thing in the morning. As you sleep, the pull of gravity is lessened and your discs are not under as much pressure. This is why you are taller in the morning than at the end of the day and also why it is the easiest time to hurt yourself. Your discs have had no pressure exerted on them during the night and are not prepared for sudden movement. Warming up increases the blood supply to the muscles, thus providing necessary oxygen. Without oxygen, cellular respiration produces lactic acid which causes muscles to cramp. This is why it is equally important to "warm down" after exercising, to continue the flow of oxygenated blood to the muscles.

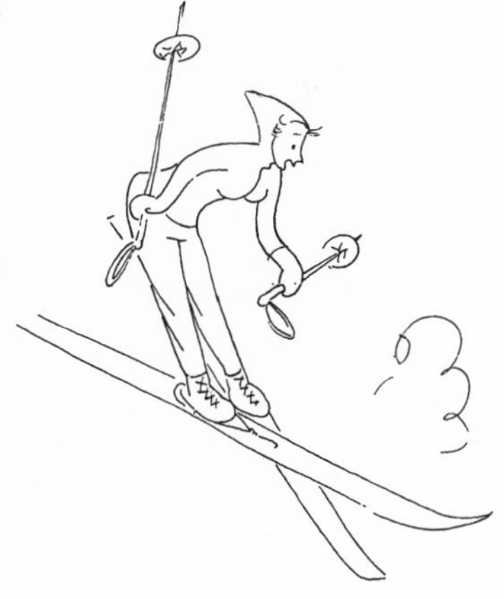

Bones, as well as muscles, benefit from exercise. When people are bedridden and stationary for long periods of time, they actually

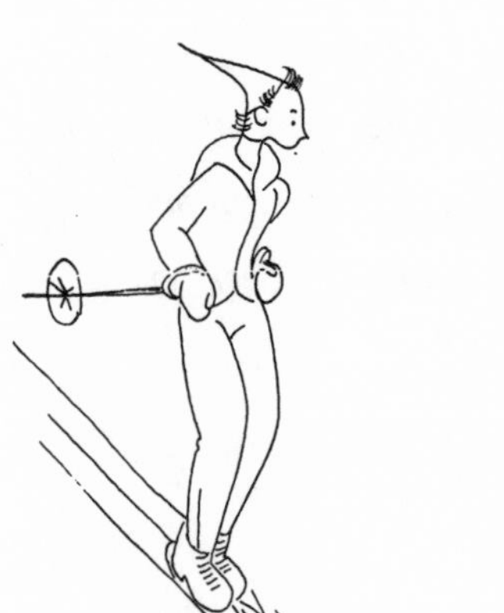

lose bone tissue and their muscles atrophy. Bones need the pull and tug of muscles to keep them healthy.

Walking, swimming (not butterfly or breast stroke), and walking in chest deep water are low-impact exercises that help build chest and thigh muscles. For non-swimmers try standing in waist deep water with your back to the wall and spell the alphabet out with one straight leg (capital or small letters – either will give your thighs and stomach muscles a good workout). You don't need to have mastered the major strokes to benefit from swimming. For a great workout of natural muscle movements, try the dogpaddle.

Walking is a wonderful exercise. It requires only supportive running shoes. (Walking shoes, advertised as such, are often less supportive than running shoes.) Make sure they fit well and bend easily at the ball of the foot. Good shoes will have a "counter" at the heel. Check by trying to bend the back of the shoe forward. Thin canvas tennis shoes bend easily and have no counter. Well made brand-name shoes almost always have a counter. Start your walking routine slowly, 5-10 minutes a day. Make a regular habit out of the daily walk. Once it has become a habit, add 5 minutes a week. If you walk 5-10 minutes the first week, 10-15 minutes the second week, *etc.*, you will be walking 40-45 minutes in a couple of months and a hour by the end of three months.

Yoga is a wonderful preventive exercise. Some orthopedists and sports doctors find that the postures and movements of yoga are among the best for keeping the back pain free. Strengthening and stretching exercises are done slowly in yoga along with a concentration on breathing. (See yoga section for specific exercises).

Perhaps the most widely known back care exercise program in the world is the YMCA program "Y's Way to a Healthy Back." Check with your local Y for classes.

§ *Get light-weight cooking pans. The cast iron stew pot, or large cast iron frying pan is heavier than you think.*

In most university towns, and in larger cities particularly on the west and east coast, you might be able to find a class in Tai Chi, a form of Chinese exercise. Tai Chi is done standing up and slowly moving, shifting your weight from position to position. These slow moving exercises help foster balance and flexiblity. They are often taught as a routine that keeps moving. Millions of elderly Chinese head to the parks in China in the early morning to do their Tai Chi for the day. It is a great exercise program for someone who has pain, has had an operation or is otherwise left out of more strenuous exercise regimes.

The last place to get helpful exercise information is your sports gym. These programs are geared to healthy people who want to get in shape, and rarely is there expert help available for the person with the problem back.

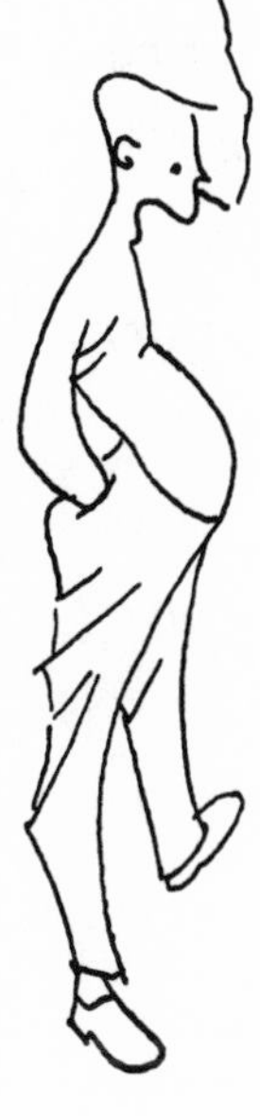

❍ SPORTS

If you led an active sport-filled life before you began to have back trouble, there is no reason you can't continue to do so with some minor adjustments. According to Augustus White's Your Aching Back, some of the sports with lowest risk of back injury include swimming (except butterfly stroke), hockey, lacrosse, tennis, skiing and tobogganing. Slightly higher risk sports include baseball, bowling, golf and jogging. Sports with the highest risk of back injury include gymnastics, football and rowing.

Keep in mind that no activity is risk free. Proper body mechanics and good overall body conditioning are crucial to healthy participation in sports. For sports like golf and baseball where twisting is a primary motion, proper technique can make all the difference between a high-risk activity and a low-risk one. If you've had a back injury, take the time to relearn the basic strokes of your sport with new attention to your back. Get coaching if necessary and learn to avoid specific high-risk moves if possible. You may want to find a Sports Medicine Specialist who is familiar with treating injuries in your particular sport.

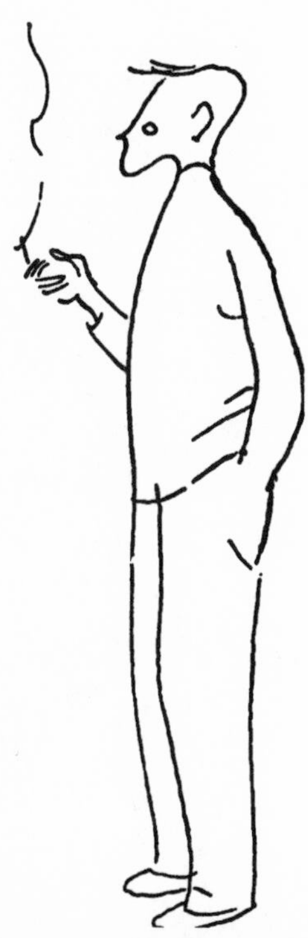

❍ HABITS

Old habits are hard to break. They take self-determination, willpower and a motivating force. You may not be able to "clean up your act" at once. So pick the one thing you've always wanted to change and then do it. Not tommorrow, or next week, but **now** is the time to change your life, for you!

Weight Loss

A healthy body weight is essential to good body mechanics. Losing those extra pounds you carry around everyday could be just the relief your back needs. Plus, you will reduce the risk of heart attack and other health problems associated with obesity.

§ *Whether it is brushing your teeth, putting on makeup or shaving, leaning into the mirror over a sink is a daily mistake likely to cause pain. Instead put one foot in front of the other and bend at the hips.*

Smoking

We all know by now that cigarette smoking is bad for your health in general, but it has a specific impact on your back as well. Smoking can produce a chronic cough which can increase stress on the abdomen and lumbar discs. Smoking can diminish the mineral content of bone, weakening it and making it more vulnerable to fractures. Smoking also decreases blood flow to the discs which can leave them undernourished. In addition, research has shown that it takes smokers longer to heal from injuries and operations. Hospitals may require that you quit smoking for a certain length of time before an operation. If you are a habitual smoker, it might also be good for your sanity to quit before entering the hospital because it is rare for hospitals to allow smoking.

Coffee

As much a part of the American way of life as the coffee break itself. Constant coffee drinking can leave you feeling jittery and nervous. The buzz that keeps you going may lull you into believing you can get more done, faster. This stressful way to live sets the stage for back trouble. Your mind is often on what you're going to do next, not on where your body is and what it is doing. If you find yourself drinking nothing but coffee all morning, try something different at lunch. Make your last cup of coffee for the day the one after dinner. Drinking coffee at 11pm is a sure way to be up all night which can only leave you tired and tense the next day. Coffee is best avoided when you're laid up with back pain. You'll drive yourself crazy drinking coffee all day with no way to expend the energy.

BACK SURGERY

What You Can Expect

Surgery is not the magic cure. Unless the condition is immediately life-threatening, one should approach surgery as a last resort. If, after weighing all the information and getting at least two medical opinions, you have decided that it would considerably improve the quality of your life, then going through with surgery may be your best option. Be aware, however, that while it may help some of your problems (sciatica, tingling, numbness), it sometimes creates new problems as well. In a large number of cases, perhaps as many as 60%, surgery did not heal chronic low back pain.

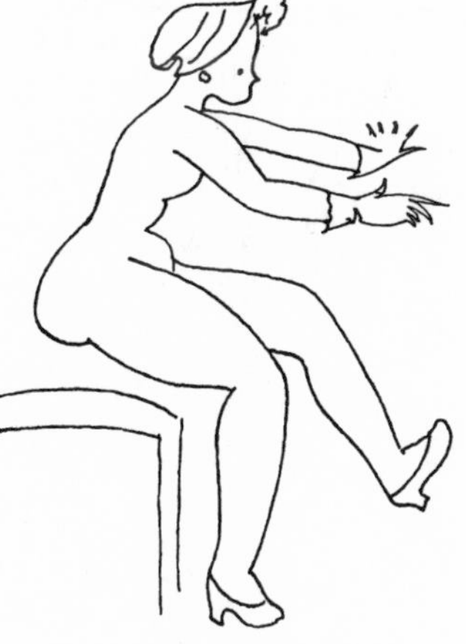

Unless you are going for a new procedure, not done elsewhere, it is best to shop around for both a surgeon and a medical facility. Usually a doctor will only have the right to perform surgery at one hospital. This means that you will also have the anesthesiologist, physical therapists, nurses and other support staff of that hospital to help you before, during and after surgery. You will want an orthopedic specialist *i.e.* one specializing in lower backs, or upper backs, or necks, *etc.* One who does 100 surgeries a year is better than one who rarely ever has to perform the kind of operation you will need.

Check out what kind of physical therapy they will suggest for you after surgery. Do they have a back school on the premises? If so, see if you can go to the back school first. Often this is enough re-education to improve your situation. Many good hospitals require patients planning surgery to attend the back school first and have found that this dramatically decreases the number of back surgeries performed. Even if you do still need surgery, a back school can teach you the skills you will need to know when you are recovering and afterward, how to move, relax and exercise. Find out if the hospital is connected to an out-patient spine center? Be wary of long in-patient physical therapy programs.

It is hard enough being in pain. Having to be your own advocate for good health care at the same time can be overwhelming. Try and go over as many questions as you might think of before going into the hospital. (See "Before Saying Yes To Surgery.") Think ahead! Try and get a clear picture of what is going to happen, how long you'll be in the hospital, how much pain there is likely to be, what the worst case scenario might be like. You may want to look into providing your own blood (autogolous transfusion) in case it is needed for transfusion. You must start looking into this procedure months in advance. Talk to your doctor about how this is done is your area. You may need to contact the hospital or the local blood bank that the hospital uses. You can also ask friends and family to give blood for your operation (this may also need to be cleared with local blood banks and the hospital months in advance). Blood banks won't accept donations from people who are anemic, ever had hepatitis, or are HIV positive.

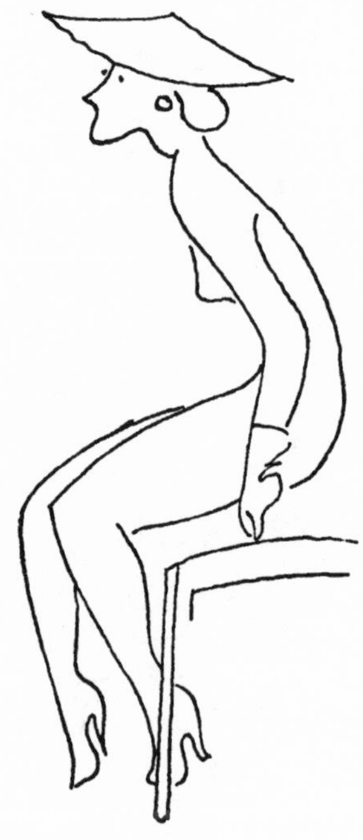

How fast you heal and recover after surgery is directly related to the condition you are in before surgery. Many surgeons may want you to lose 20 pounds first, if you can, or gain 20, if you are seriously underweight. The sooner you can stop smoking the better. Start thinking about general conditioning well in advance of your surgery.

Let your friends and family know before you decide on dates. Visits in the hospital are a welcome relief from the sterile atmosphere and rigors of pain. See if someone can be there in the hospital when you come out of surgery. It might be hard to have family and friends see you at your worst, but you will be relieved at the sight of a familiar face in those first difficult hours.

Before you enter the hospital, make the necessary arrangements for when you come out. You will need to think about both who will take care of you, and who will take care of those things that you will be unable to attend to. Now is the time to swallow your pride and realize that you will need to ask for help. People are busy, but if you can work out what you need ahead of time, plans can be made that work for everyone. If you are the type who is always helping others, then you know how rewarding that feeling is. Let others experience that same good feeling helping you.

"The rate of lumbar spine surgery in the United States is three to eight times higher than in most European countries, suggesting that it may be overused."
— *Annals of Internal Medicine*

If you're lucky enough to have a choice, then you need to decide where you are going to be. Being at home, in familiar surroundings with spouse, children and/or pets nearby, can be very comforting. But your home may need some rearranging or you may need to plan on staying with a relative or friend. Ideally, your bedroom and bathroom should be on the main floor, with no stairs to climb. Most importantly, a telephone should be near your bed in case anything happens.

Be aware that you will probably be spending a good part of the first several months after surgery in bed and at first, probably in a good deal of pain. Every little task, even rolling over in bed, may seem enormously difficult. You may need help getting to the bathroom. Is there someone who can be home with you all day, especially for the first two weeks (or the first month after a spinal fusion)? Can you afford to hire someone to be with you when family or friends can't be there? If you're not so fortunate to have a friend or relative who can come and help for 2 weeks to get your meals and answer the door, maybe a key can be left for friends to let themselves in.

Meals should be planned (who will make them, or bring them over, who will heat and bring them to you.) Your household chores should be seen to (who will do the food shopping, the laundry, take out the garbage, clean the house, take care of the kids, animals, water the plants, get the paper off the porch, *etc.*). A television should be up high, so you can see it laying on your back in bed (here is the best use for a remote). A small tape player and tapes, or radio can provide music and information. A pitcher for water or a pump thermos with your favorite beverage, kleenex, paper and pen should be nearby. It is very difficult to hold a book above your head while your on your back. You may want to look into Books on Tape. It's a great gift for the bedridden; some public libraries also carry them. Everything you need should be within your reach. Surround yourself with those things and people that will help the healing process go faster, your favorite pictures, blankets, bolsters, pillows, *etc.*

"Operations on bones and joints almost always are followed by rehabilitative and physical therapy to ease your limb or joint back into use and shape. Having your surgery done at a major center improves your chances of getting the best in postoperative care; most have on-site physical therapy facilities and equipment. The equipment should be up-to-date and new, and the physical-therapy staff should be forthcoming about details of the program and how long it should last in the wake of an operation of your type."

— *U.S. News and World Report*

Your support group of family and friends should be trained to ask, "How Can I Help?" Don't allow them to make the mistake, all too common in our society, of believing that the "invalid" is in-valid. Nothing will destroy your morale more than having people ask each other what you want for dinner when you're lying there awake, fully conscious. Train them to ask. And don't allow them to determine your priorities. If the house is a mess and you want the garden weeded, let them know that that's the best way they can help you. Make sure you let your needs be known.

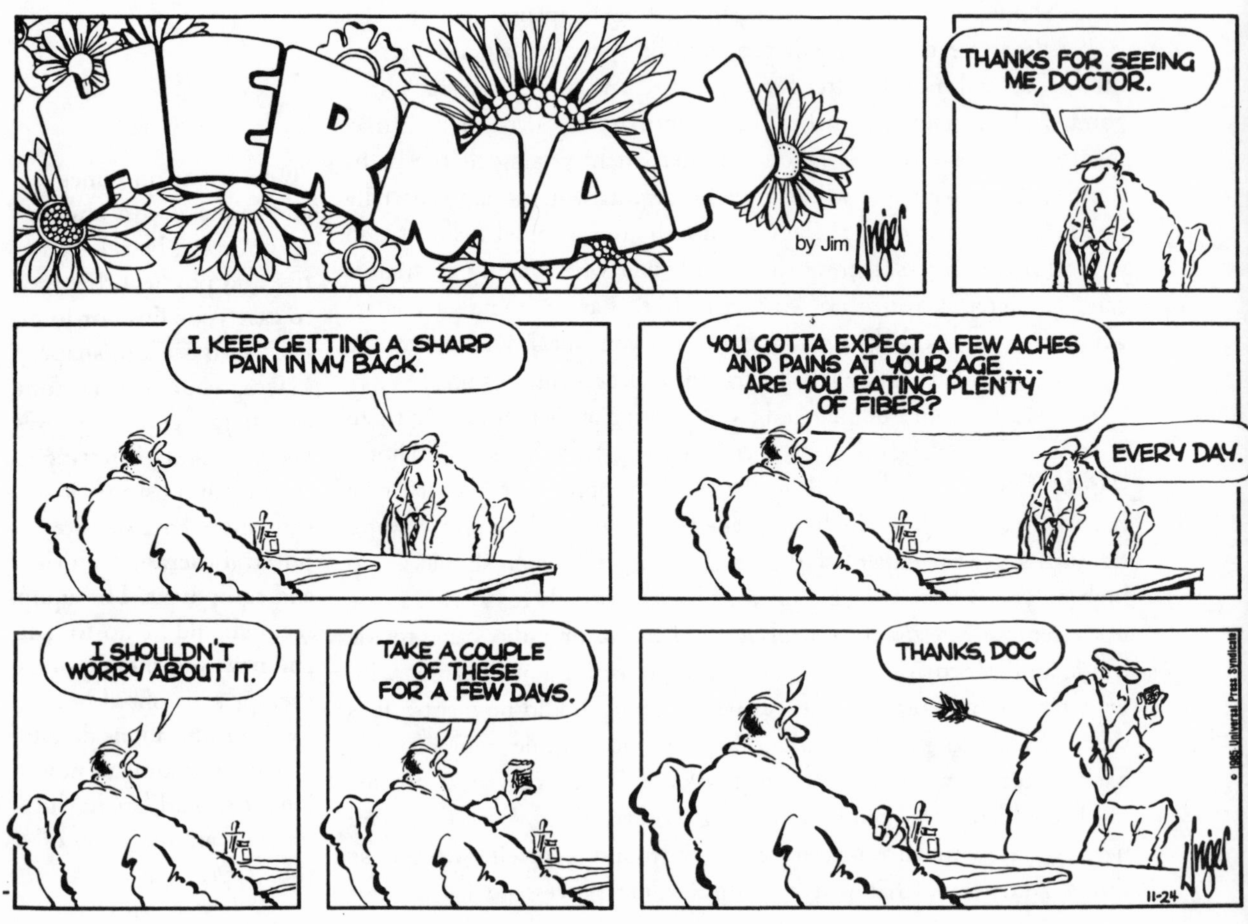
HERMAN
by Jim Unger
THANKS FOR SEEING ME, DOCTOR.
I KEEP GETTING A SHARP PAIN IN MY BACK.
YOU GOTTA EXPECT A FEW ACHES AND PAINS AT YOUR AGE.... ARE YOU EATING PLENTY OF FIBER?
EVERY DAY.
I SHOULDN'T WORRY ABOUT IT.
TAKE A COUPLE OF THESE FOR A FEW DAYS.
THANKS, DOC
© 1985 Universal Press Syndicate
Unger
11-24

BEFORE SAYING "YES" TO SURGERY

Questions to Ask Before Entering the Hospital

By Lawrence Galton

By asking the right questions, you or those you love will get first-rate medical care.

1. Unless it's an emergency, be sure to get a second expert opinion. Most health insurers will pay for a second opinion, and many will now pay for a third consultation if the first two doctors offer conflicting advice.
2. If you have difficulty locating another specialist, call the Second Surgical Opinion Hotline in Washington, DC, toll-free: 800-638-6833. Other good sources for referrals: your county medical society, a local medical school or state hospital, and friends who have already undergone the procedure.
3. Avoid repeating x-rays and other diagnostic tests by asking the first-opinion doctor to forward your medical records to the physician(s) you select for further consultations.
4. Carefully check out each surgeon's qualifications. Ask where he or she received medical training or write to Physician Biographic Records, American Medical Association, 515 N. State St., Chicago, IL 60610, for biographical information. Include a self-addressed, stamped envelope and allow three weeks for a response.
5. Be sure the doctor is licensed by the state. In addition, a board-certified physician has passed special examinations specifically

§ *Take your time – if it's not a matter of life and death, it doesn't have to be done today.*

to perform surgery. "The Directory of Medical Specialists" at your local library can provide this information.

6. Determine whether there is a non-surgical alternative to your operation. Can you be helped with medications, special diet or by other means without resorting to surgery?
7. Ask whether any of the newer surgical "knifeless" techniques – laser surgery (for procedures involving the eyes), cryosurgery (for removing skin tumors), arthroscopy (for elbow or knee joints) or balloon angioplasty (for opening up narrowed arteries), for example – might be appropriate in your case.
8. Question the surgeon about the consequences, if any, should you decide not to have the operation or delay it to some future date.
9. Ask about any risks and/or complications that may accompany the procedure. Any competent surgeon will discuss these factors with you.
10. Ask how often the surgeon performs this procedure. Generally there is less risk with a doctor who does an operation on a regular basis.
11. Try to determine the surgeon's personal success (and failure) rate by questioning your family physician and others who may know of the specialist by reputation.
12. Ask to be told exactly what will occur during the operation. It's reasonable to request that answers be rephrased if something isn't clear.
13. Ask which hospital (or hospitals) the surgeon is affiliated with. Will you feel comfortable there? Is it convenient to your home? This information may help you when it comes time to narrow down your choice of doctors.
14. Ask the surgeon if he or she will perform the operation personally, or if it will be done by a resident-in-training under the surgeon's supervision. Then ask yourself how you feel about that.
15. Ask if the surgeon will follow your case after the operation. Will you be turned over to an associate afterward? If so, is that acceptable to you?
16. Find out what type of anesthetic you are likely to have. Then ask if the anesthesiologist can visit you before the operation to answer any questions you may have.

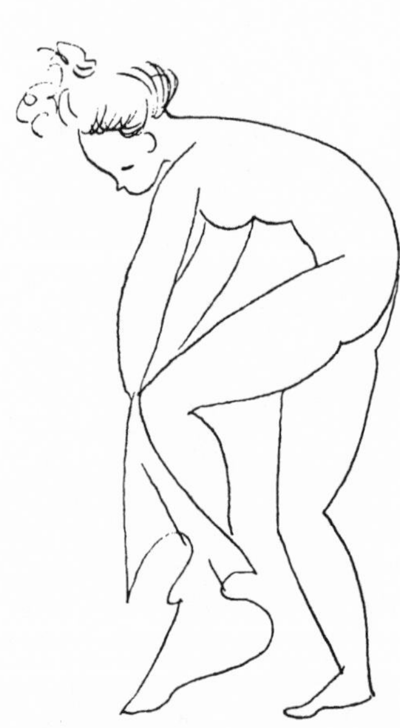

17. If you cannot be anesthetized for medical reasons or do not tolerate chemical anesthesia well, check out a new but growing alternative: hypnosis, or hypnosis in conjunction with anesthesia. In the hands of a trained technician, hypnosis is also useful for relieving anxiety and alleviating pain. To locate a member of the American Society of Clinical Hypnosis near where you live, send a self-addressed, stamped envelope to 2200 E. Devon Avenue, Suite 291, Des Plaines, IL 60018.
18. Consider that hospitals are often short of staff over weekends and during major holiday periods. If your surgery is elective, can you schedule around this?
19. Be sure to find out all the fees that are involved. Are postsurgical follow-up visits included?
20. Find out if the operation can be done on an outpatient basis or as same-day surgery. It may be possible to have any necessary tests performed the day before, check into the hospital or ambulatory care center on the day of surgery, then go home later the same day.
21. Ask about donating your own blood in advance of the procedure. Should you need a transfusion, the remote but possible complications that can arise from donor blood (hepatitis, for example) can be avoided.
22. Take as much time as you need to read and understand the forms you are asked to sign at the hospital admitting office. And don't allow anyone to intimidate you if you have questions or need more time.
23. Ask your doctor when he or she expects to be "making rounds" or visiting you in the hospital. Then be prepared: Write down any questions, problems or concerns that you wish to discuss.
24. Ask if you will be restricted in any way once you are discharged from the hospital. How long before you can return to your regular activities, household duties, job or volunteer work?
25. Find out in advance of the surgery whether you'll need to arrange for someone to help you with household chores while you are recuperating at home. For how long?
26. Ask if you should have a friend or relative drive you home from the hospital. Sometimes drowsiness, weakness or muscle incoordination can linger for several days.

§ *Get an automatic car, the next time you replace your old one. Working the three foot pedals on a manual transmission puts a lot of wear and tear on the lower back.*

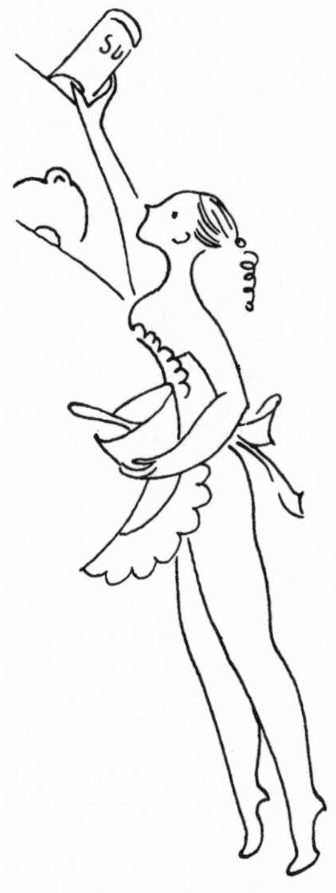

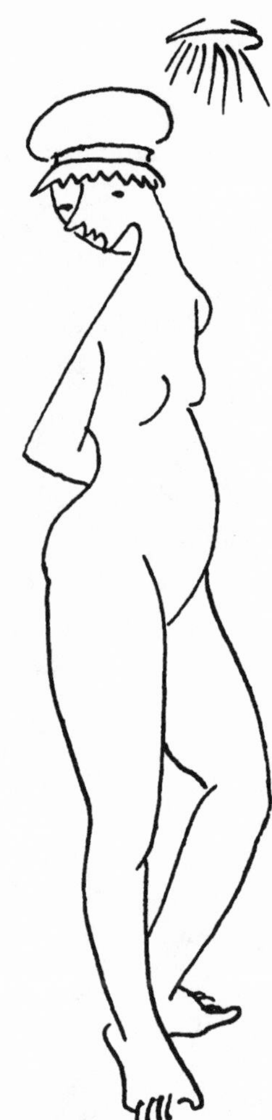

§ *Get tools and machines that are lightweight, yet powerful.*

27. Ask the nurse or doctor to suggest ways to minimize the common postoperative discomforts of turning in bed, breathing and coughing. Carry out the maneuvers about 30 minutes after you receive a pain reliever. Another help: Clutch a pillow to your abdomen when you cough.
28. Ask to see the hospital dietitian about personalizing your menu, if possible. With your doctor's consent, some hospitals can provide meals geared toward your particular preferences.
29. Ask if it's possible for you to administer your own pain relief. In some hospitals, a machine can be hooked into the intravenous tubing that will deliver a controlled amount of painkilling drug directly into the bloodstream with a simple push of a button.

    It has been observed that patients who self-administer their medication actually require less painkilling drugs than when it's given by hospital staff.
30. If patient-controlled pain relief is not available and you are very uncomfortable, discuss adjusting the medication to meet your needs.
31. If your operation leaves you with an unsightly scar, ask whether plastic surgery can minimize the scar.
32. Ask your doctor to write out any postsurgery instructions: diet, exercise restrictions, medication schedule, *etc.*, so there's no misunderstanding about what you should and should not do.
33. Find out what specific symptoms signal a potential problem and indicate that a need to call the doctor. Find out when you should return to have sutures removed, if that pertains to you.
34. Check your hospital bill carefully. In 1984 and early 1985, one company that audits hospital bills for insurers and self-insured employers found errors that resulted in overcharges in 97 percent of the bills they examined.

About the Author

Lawrence Galton, formerly a columnist for *Family Circle* magazine, specializes in medicine and health. His book, *Med Tech* is published by Harper & Row. This article first appeared in the October 15, 1985 issue of *Family Circle*.

"Only about 1 percent of all back problems require surgery. . . . Surgery is most successful when a patient has:

• Numbness or a loss of reflex in one or both legs.

• Pain radiating down one or both legs when nerves in the back are stretched.

• A damaged disc shown on an MRI image. If all three symptoms are present, surgery works over 90 percent of the time. But in only two of the three symptoms, surgery relieves the pain in only 60 percent of cases."

– Joseph Alper,
Washington Post Health

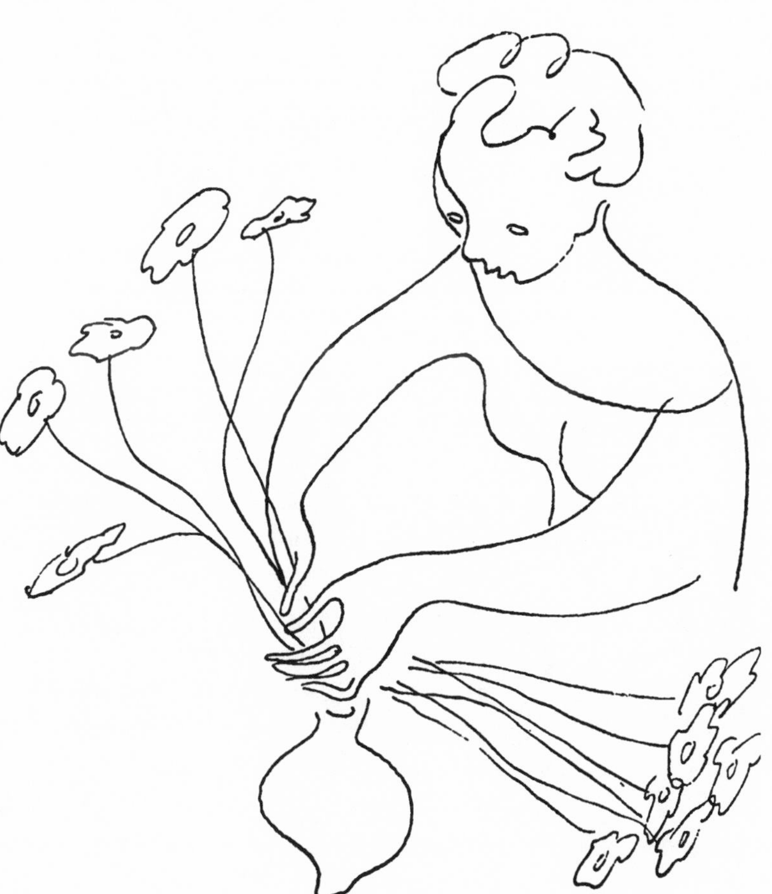

TYPES OF BACK SURGERY

❍ LAMINECTOMIES/DISCECTOMIES

A removal of some portion of the disc. An incision is made in your back (or through your front) and a small area of the vertebrae is removed (laminectomy) or the part of the disc impinging on the nerves is cut away (discectomy). This operation has been done for more than 50 years.

"Approximately 200,000 back surgeries will be performed this year in the United States alone; of these, 85 percent will be successful to a significant degree. Even so, a third of all back operations are followed by a second surgery. And what about the 15 percent that prove unsuccessful? That's 30,000 people who endured the anguish of back surgery only to find no relief from their pain – or to find that their pain had worsened."
– Edward Abraham, *Freedom From Back Pain*

❍ FUSION

Replacement of a disc with bone taken from a donor, or from behind the front crest of the hip bone. The idea is that living bone will grow over the area in your back and "fuse" the back. It may get rid of sciatica for all or some time, but many complain that back pain is still there after surgery. It is an extremely painful operation which usually requires at least a week in a hospital and about 6 months to heal. The success rate for using this type of surgery to cure simple low back pain is low.

❍ CHEMONUCLEOLYSIS

Chymopapain is an enzyme derived from papaya. A small amount, one-third of a teaspoonful, is injected into the problem disc while the patient is under general anesthesia and under an x-ray machine. The enzyme is supposed to dissolve the nucleus of the disc. Although it reached its heyday in the mid to late 1970's, it was only approved for use by the FDA in 1982. A couple of years later it had fallen out of favor due to its adverse side affects. Only in the last couple of years

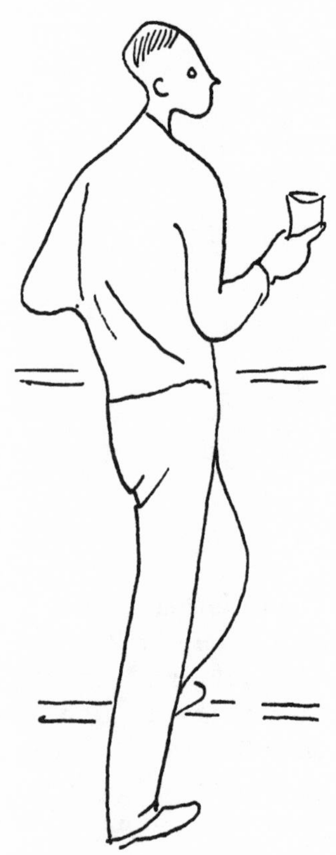

has interest been cautiously growing. It is significantly less expensive than a laminectomy and the patient usually recovers more quickly (although there have been reported cases of severe back pain for 3-12 weeks). Some past side affects have been nerve damage (including paralysis), allergic reactions (including anaphylactic shock), itching, dizziness, headaches, cerebral hemorrhage, spinal pain and nausea. Make sure the doctor tests for allergic reaction before injecting the enzyme into your spine. Papaya-based proteins are so widely used in meat tenderizers, papaya enzyme pills, beer, and cosmetics, that many people could have developed sensitivities to it without knowing. Also, it has not been proven that chymopapain only dissolves the nucleus of the disk. There are reports that it can dissolve the whole disc leaving bone to rub against bone.

Don't let this dissuade you. The important thing is to get a second opinion. Chemonucleolysis is not a cure for low back pain, rather an alternative to laminectomies, discectomies, and fusions. Success rates range from 60-75 percent.

Remember, many of the early procedures were performed by inexperienced doctors who were not sufficiently trained in its use. Some doctors probably did less than 5-10 in their lives. If you're really interested, find a doctor who has a proven track record of successful results. There are many former back pain sufferers who honestly believe it was the answer for them.

❍ MICROSURGERY

"95 percent of the neurological complications associated with the earlier use of chymopapain stemmed from faulty injections, including accidentally shooting the drug into the spinal canal, by doctors who had treated fewer than 10 patients."
– Warren E. Leary, *Freedom from Back Pain*

Surgery for laminectomies using a microscope so that the incision site need only be an inch long. Pain is often less because the incision is smaller. If the doctor is sure of the exact location where the disc is impinging on the nerve, this may be the answer. Sometimes, though, it is just a little to the right or left, up or down and thus the limitations are a hinderance. These surgeries are sometimes considered failures because symptoms reappear due to missed parts of disks.

Microsurgery has many advantages. Nerves to the spinal muscle aren't cut. Ligaments to the spine aren't cut. Damage to tissue is far less. Patients feel their body hasn't been invaded as radically which acts as a psychological aid to healing. Less postoperative medication is needed and hospital stays can be reduced.

THE PAPERWORK MAZE

Back Pain and Disability Insurance

By Kelly Dunn and Jennifer Atkins

An individual's ability to function in all areas, including at work, may be significantly limited by back pain. If back problems prevent you from maintaining your employment, you may find yourself experiencing severe financial hardship and in need of assistance. If you are a member of a private disability insurance plan, you should immediately contact your insurance company to obtain details regarding your coverage. If you do not have private disability insurance, you may be eligible for one (or more) of the available state and Federal disability benefits programs.

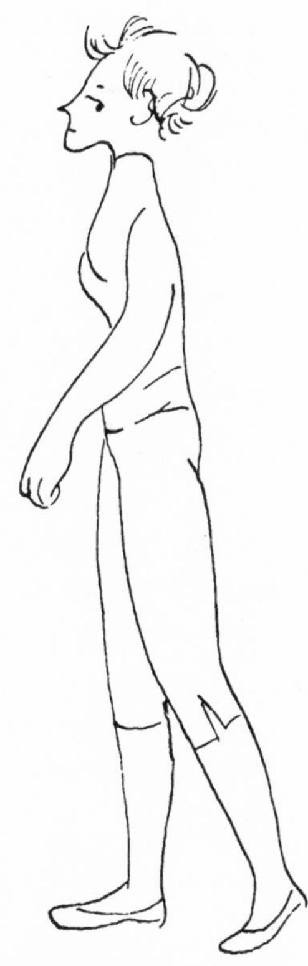

The focus of this section is Social Security benefits, the largest nationwide, Federally funded disability benefits program. Social Security is a long-term disability program, designed for people who are, or expect to be, disabled for at least 12 months. You should also be familiar, however, with other state programs which may be available to you: State Disability Insurance and Workers' Compensation. A brief outline of these programs is also provided.

Social Security benefits, State disability benefits and Workers' Compensation benefits are each based on your inability to work. You should be aware that three additional programs may be available to you which do not require that you be disabled: General Assistance (Welfare), Aid to Families with Dependent Children (AFDC), and Unemployment Insurance. While a discussion of these programs is beyond the scope of this article, please note that General Assistance and AFDC have very stringent financial and resource requirements which must be met to establish eligibility. The Unemployment Insurance program requires that you certify that you are able-bodied and are actively seeking employment, assertions which are in direct opposition to the statements you must make to qualify for disability benefits. If you are in need of immediate financial assistance after you have stopped working due to a disability, you are advised to apply for either State Disability Insurance benefits or General Assistance/AFDC, if you meet the eligibility criteria for those programs.

"In workers under 45 years of age, back problems are the most common cause of disability."
– Arthritis Foundation

❍ STATE DISABILITY INSURANCE

Most States administer a disability insurance program for people who are temporarily unable to work (12 months or less). The benefits are earnings-based; a percentage of your earnings is withheld from your paycheck for your State Disability Insurance. Once you have paid into the program a specified minimum amount for the required number of months you will be insured. The amount of your benefit depends upon the level of your past income. Benefits may be paid for up to 12 months, but generally will not extend beyond 12 months.

You should file your claim for State Disability benefits as soon as you are unable to go to work. Benefits may be denied if not filed in a timely manner. You are likely to be awarded these benefits if you are unable to go to work and your physician is willing to certify (on the appropriate form) that your medical condition is disabling. Your employer is required to provide you with information regarding State Disability Insurance benefits, including the telephone number and address of the office in your area.

❍ WORKERS' COMPENSATION

Each state also administers a Workers' Compensation benefits program. To qualify, you must have suffered an injury on the job. You need not be off work for any minimum period of time. Benefits may also be available for partial disability. That is, you do not need to prove that you were rendered completely disabled by the injury. Other non-monetary benefits may also be available to you. These include medical treatment for the injury and vocational rehabilitation services.

You can obtain a Workers' Compensation claim form from your employer or from the local Workers' Compensation appeals board. *You should notify your employer immediately in writing that an injury has occurred.* If the claim is not filed within the time allowed by the Workers' Compensation law in your state, it will be barred. If a question arises as to the period for filing a claim, contact an attorney who specializes in Workers' Compensation claims. Again, if you decide to pursue a claim, you may obtain further information regarding the process from your employer. Employers are required to provide pertinent information to their employees regarding the state agency that regulates Workers' Compensation claims. If you are not satisfied with the way your claim is being handled, you should seriously consider consulting an attorney.

"In workers under 45 years of age, back problems are the most common cause of disability."
– Arthritis Foundation

❍ SOCIAL SECURITY DISABILITY BENEFITS

Social Security Disability Benefits are only available to individuals who are, or expect to be, disabled for a period of at least 12 months. You need not – and should not – wait until you have been disabled 12 months before applying. If you expect your disability to last 12 months, you should apply immediately. In determining whether you are disabled, the Social Security Administration ("SSA") considers whether you can perform any of the kinds of work that you have engaged in during the previous 15 years or, if not, whether you have the capacity to engage in less strenuous forms of work. The SSA is not concerned with and does not consider whether the job pays significantly less than you are used to or whether job openings are available in the region in which you live. SSA is only concerned with whether you have the physical and mental capacity to work.

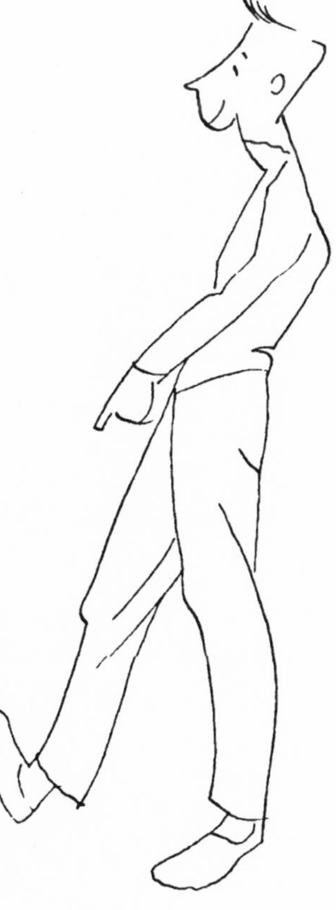

Two separate but related disability benefit programs are administered by the SSA. The first of these programs, Disability Insurance Benefits (SSDI), is earnings-based, like state disability insurance. It is essentially an insurance program available to people who have paid into Social Security during their working years. To qualify for SSDI, you must be disabled and you must have worked 20 out of the 40 quarters prior to becoming disabled (roughly 5 of the last 10 years). The other program, Supplemental Security Income (SSI), is a welfare program providing benefits for all disabled individuals regardless of whether they have paid any money into Social Security. To qualify for SSI, you must be disabled and you must meet strict income/resource requirements.

"In people aged 45 to 64 years of age, back pain is third only to heart disease and arthritis and rheumatism as a cause of chronic disability."
— David Borenstein, *Current Science*

If you apply for Social Security benefits because of your back pain, be forewarned that there are certain difficulties peculiar to claims based on back pain. Social Security is a medical program; a finding of disability requires "objective" medical findings (positive test results) as well as your subjective complaints of pain. However, x-ray examinations often fail to reveal the injury that causes back pain, or the pain may be disproportionate to the objective findings. While there are more sophisticated tests which may detect the cause of discomfort, *e.g.*, MRI, CT scan, and EMG, these tests are costly and usually are not performed unless complaints of pain have persisted for a long time and are consistent with a type of injury not likely to appear on x-rays. Furthermore, the effect of other factors contributing to back pain cannot be objectively verified. These factors include obesity, poor posture, stress and depression.

There are several steps you can take to strengthen your claim. First, try to obtain consistent and regular medical treatment for your back discomfort. Beware: SSA does not give the same weight to treatment records of a chiropractor as they do to those of an MD. If your only treatment is from a chiropractor, there is a strong likelihood your claim will be denied. If chiropractic, or other non-traditional medical treatment, is your treatment of choice, consider supplementing it with regular visits to an MD, preferably one who is accepting of non-medical alternatives. Secondly, document your impairment with tests that will reveal the cause of your pain. In some settings, this may require some persistence on your part to get appropriate tests run. Try to get your practitioner to understand that you need objective evidence in order to receive support. Thirdly, be sure your physician is aware of all the problems and symptoms you are having with your back, not just the main difficulty. For example, if you have occasional tingling sensations radiating down a leg, make sure you report that to your physician. Fourthly, you should submit corroborating evidence such as statements from friends or family members regarding your back pain and resulting limitations. Finally, provide detailed information on your application regarding adjustments you have had to make in your life as a result of your pain, *e.g.*, you sleep on the floor, you do dishes while sitting on a stool, *etc.*

Applying for either SSDI or SSI and pursuing the process to its end can become very involved and take in excess of two years before benefits are awarded. The process can be lengthy because frequently claims are denied both at the initial application stage and at the first level of appeal (the reconsideration stage). There are several reasons for the initial denials, ranging from a claimant's inadequate documentation to the SSA's bureaucratic backlog and failure to properly apply its own regulations. After being denied twice, people often experience frustration and depression. It is very difficult to be unable to perform your usual employment, to live with little money, and to have the government repeatedly tell you that you are healthy and can go back to work. However, if you do persist and appeal your reconsidera-tion denial, your patience is more likely to be rewarded at the third stage of the process when you are given the opportunity to present your case at a hearing.

§ *If the pain is really bad, sleep on your back with pillows under your knees, or try sleeping on your side with a pillow between your drawn up knees. This helps to stop your pelvis from rolling foreward as your knees meet. (It might seem strange at first but this works.)*

The majority of claims (approximately 60%) are granted at the hearing stage of the process. Accordingly, it is of vital importance that you begin the application process at the earliest possible date and that each step in the process be completed in a timely manner. If it is necessary for you to go to hearing, you should contact an attorney or representative who specializes in Social Security law to help you prepare and present your case.

Negotiating the paperwork maze outlined in this article is often demoralizing and depressing, particularly when you are experiencing physical and/or mental distress. However, the process is likely to be significantly less exasperating if you are aware of the many hurdles you are likely to face and how to overcome them. Hopefully, your benefits will be awarded when you first apply and you can then devote your time to caring for yourself and learning how to live with your back condition.

About the Authors:

Kelly Dunn is an attorney and Executive Director at The Hawkins Center of Law and Services for the Disabled. Jennifer Atkins is a Staff Attorney with The Hawkins Center. The Hawkins Center, located in Richmond, California, provides legal representation and support services to applicants seeking Social Security disability benefits.

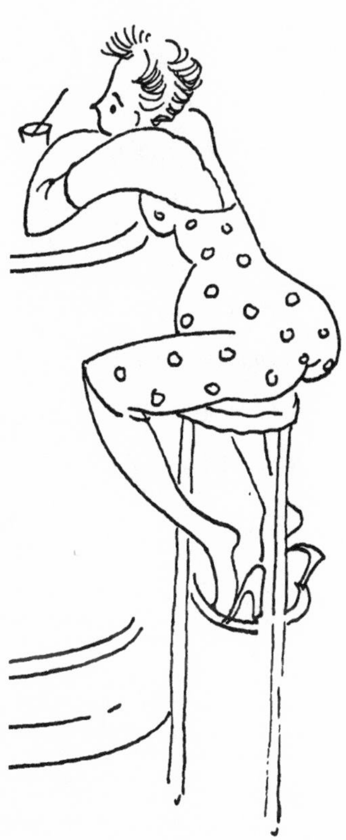

WHAT IF NOTHING WORKS

Tending to back care problems immediately when they come up is the best way to shorten the agony of the experience. (See the First 48 Hours section). Ignoring the problem will not make it go away, and stay away. Ultimately, you might find that your situation will become worse because the back pain will return to plague you again and again.

If your back is not responding to bedrest, see your health care worker. Sometimes back pain can be caused by problems with other internal organs: kidneys, liver, *etc.* The peace of mind you'll receive from ruling out more serious problems is worth the expense and trouble. If you are like 80-90% of all Americans, you have "garden variety" low back pain, but proper diagnosis can be crucial for the other 10-20%. If the prescribed treatment by one practitioner does not improve your situation, visit another type of practitioner. If you went to an orthopedist, go see an internist or chiropractor. Different practitioners are trained to look for, and therefore they find, different things.

Surveys of what works suggest that, ultimately, the therapies that work the best are those where the patient is actively involved: yoga, traditional exercises, fitness instruction. If overworked or improperly worked muscles are causing the problem, then the recovery is primarily up to you. If your doctor or physical therapist recommends an exercise program or physical therapy, stick to it religiously. You must train yourself to set aside half an hour a day, with no interruptions, to do these exercises in a slow, calm manner and to learn to stop if there is an increase in pain.

§ *Sit up straight on couches and use pillows or bolsters to fill in the area behind your back.*

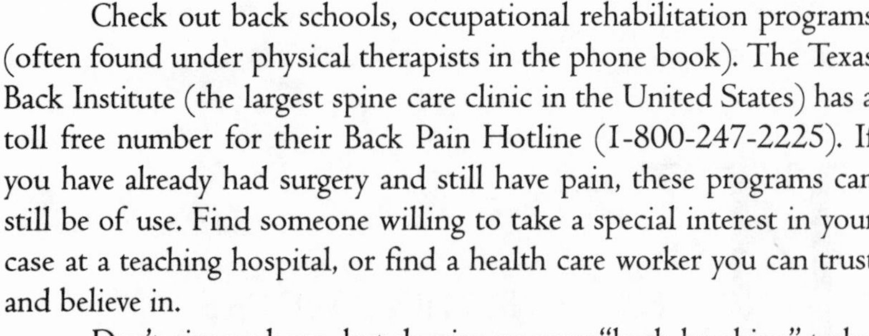

Check out back schools, occupational rehabilitation programs (often found under physical therapists in the phone book). The Texas Back Institute (the largest spine care clinic in the United States) has a toll free number for their Back Pain Hotline (1-800-247-2225). If you have already had surgery and still have pain, these programs can still be of use. Find someone willing to take a special interest in your case at a teaching hospital, or find a health care worker you can trust and believe in.

§ *There is a special Backsaver rake made now. There is also a Backsaver snow shovel. However, a yard full of leaves or walks on a corner lot are better left to someone without back problems.*

Don't give up hope, but do give up your "back-breaking" tasks. Relax more often and do away with as much stress in your life as possible. Massages and hot tubs may relax you enough to keep on going. Get involved on a level you can manage: a less demanding job, part-time work, or whatever interests you that you can handle. There is nothing worse than lots of time on your hands with nothing to think about but your back, the bills, and worrying about the future. It is an extremely stressful situation. Those around you may not know what you are going through. Talk it out with your spouse, family or friends. Let your needs and frustrations be known, but don't become a victim of back pain. It will help no one, least of all you, if you complain all day. Even in pain programs there is often a limit set as to how much time is devoted to the discussion of pain.

Perhaps your back is trying to tell you something: Is it that, in your determination to get back in shape, you're overexerting yourself? Is it that you've been slouching since your teenage years? Or pushing yourself with long lists of errands when you're tired from sitting at a computer all day? Or is it that you've been strong as an ox all your life and you've never given a thought to your back? Perhaps you've been attentive to the large things – like using care when lifting heavy objects – while ignoring the small ones – like leaning over the sink when you brush your teeth. Most people with back problems don't have a fantastically exciting story (of twisting the wrong way while cliff diving in Acapulco) to explain what happened. In fact, most people have no idea how their back got to this point.

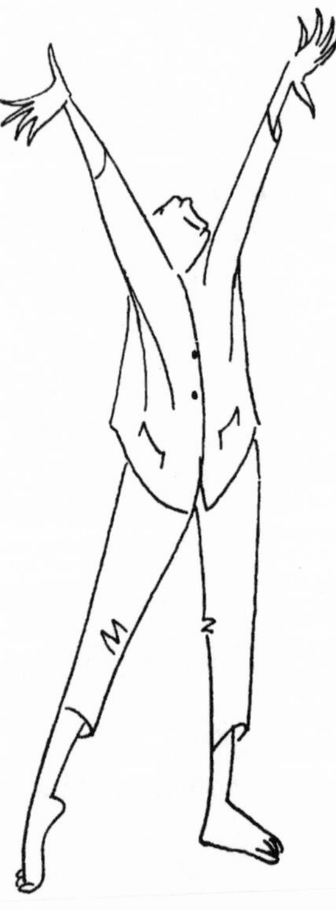

Take a good look at your life. Is the boss on your back all the time? Your spouse a pain in your neck? Though this seems overly simplistic, it can be a reason for your back pain. What is it you need to work out? Examine your life in detail, including all your past injuries. In the worst pain, the memories often come flooding back of all the times the kids at school pulled the chair out from under you and laughed when your tailbone hit the floor.

All too often the doctors say, "we've done all we can, you'll have to live with pain." But each year more advances are made in medicine, and more information is available. Keep your eyes and ears open for new information about both old and new methods. Keep in mind that just because something is the latest way to treat back pain, it doesn't mean it is the only way or the one that will work for you. It seems that in different years, different methods were the way to go. Talk to those you know. If 85% of Americans will suffer back pain in their lifetimes, chances are good that those around you have had some experience with a similar situation. Look into pain treatment centers. They can help you learn the skills you need to manage your pain, physically and emotionally.

§ *Get the best seat for the job: A bar stool for ironing, so you don't have to stoop. Ergonomically designed chairs for the workplace. Or good back cushions.*

In trying to overcome the agony of chronic pain, the support of the family and close friends cannot be underestimated. Family and friends that are intolerant of the patient's limitations or overprotective of the patient can be equally damaging to the back pain sufferer's recovery. The patient needs encouragement and support in order to do a little more each day.

You need to recognize that there is a solution for you if you are willing to take control, ask questions, and seek it out. Whether you decide on a back school, work hardening program, sports medicine rehabilitation program or a pain program, remember that each patient is an individual. No one program will work for everyone. Whatever works for you, is the right one.

You don't have to be a victim of back pain.

RESOURCES

❍ CATALOGS

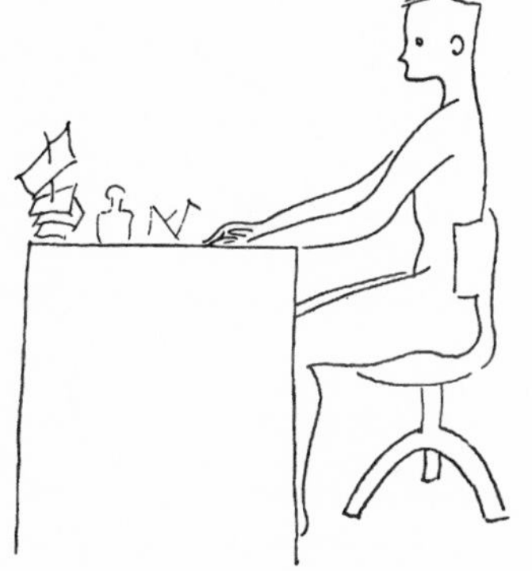

Remember that being pain-free and feeling good about yourself doesn't require a lot of consumer goods. There are some tools, though, that can make life much easier: a good back cushion, a reaching tool, a light-weight inexpensive step stool (that looks good enough to keep and use in your home), a grab bar for your shower, back cloths or back brushes for showers, long-handled shoe horns. If you work out of your home, you may want to invest in an excellent ergonomically designed chair.

❍ SPECIALTY BACK STORES

Backsaver Products Co., 53 Jeffrey Ave., Holliston, MA 01746. Call 1-800-251-2225 for a catalog. Specializing in a wide variety of chairs, the only complete living room set seen, work surfaces, back cushions, a portable bedboard and orthopedic pillow as well as the Say Goodbye to Back Pain Video.

Back Designs, 614 Grand Ave., Oakland, CA 94610. 510-451-6600. A spinal health and retail store founded by a physical therapist. Ergonomic chairs and portable sitting supports are matched to individuals based on their seated activities, physical characteristics, and comfort preferences. They also offer neck pillows, massage tools, books, and exercise equipment, including gymnastic balls. A catalog and product selection guide is available for a small charge.

The Back Shop, 125 Ocean View Boulevard, In the American Tin Cannery, Pacific Grove, CA 93950. 1-800-444-2919. Call for a

§ *If you're just reading a novel on the couch after dinner put a couple of pillows on your lap on which to rest your elbows. You'll be amazed at how much less your neck and shoulders will hurt at the end of the week.*

free catalog. They have chairs, massage chairs, automatic massage table, massage vibrators, massage cushions, back cushions, auto and truck headrests, therapeutic pillows, home seating, office chairs and equipment, footstools, desktops, copy holders, a great portable lightweight and inexpensive slant board, phone holders, massage equipment (for self massage, books, tapes, table, cushions), hot and cold wraps, cervical aids, reading aid, sleep supports, books, Say Goodbye to Back Pain video tape, inversion slant board, bath mats, lift chair, gym bar, stomach exerciser, stadium chair, headache pillow, prenatal care pillow.

Bodycare, Inc. 315 Gilmer Ferry Road, Ballground, GA 30107, 1-800-858-9888 (out of state), 1-404-735-4897 in state. Call for their flyers on cervical pillows and lumbar cushions.

Back Store by Mail, 12 North Diamond Street, C2, PO Box 528, Greenville, PA 16125. Call toll free 1-800-451-9363 for a catalog. They carry a molded car seat, Back Pain Relief video, moist heat pack, Sex and Back Pain booklet, inflatable travel pillow, tooth brush holder for the tub, industrial back support, knee support, a go anywhere back support (Nada-Chair), Craftseat (for jobs that require kneeling), back support, a reheatable heat pad, a reusable cold pack, orthopaedically designed insoles.

❍ COMPANIES for hard to find items

North Coast Medical, Inc. 450 Salmar Ave., Campbell, CA 95008 NC28664 Sock and Stocking Aid and the Matey Reaching Aid

Lumex, 100 Spence St., Bay Shore, NY 11706 product No. 6490 Versa-height toilet seat, and series 4000 Grab Bars for installation in the shower.

❍ GREAT GENERAL CATALOGS that have some handy items

Alsto's Handy Helpers, PO Box 1267, Galesburg, IL 61401.Call toll-free 1-800-447-0048 for a free catalog. Long handled brush that attaches to a garden hose for cleaning outside windows, E-Z reacher, strong shop ladders, loading ramps for vans and trucks, a 3 wheeled garden scoot, giant snow rake (over 21") for cleaning snow off roofs, the moveable hospital/tray table, an adjustable lumbar spine support cushion, inflatable drivers seat, Hi-Lo allows you to water hanging plants by a retractable device, long-handled trowel, a tool to help plant bulbs without bending, garden carts, space saving wall arms, and many more useful tools for home and garden.

§ Stay away from bending over a low oven. Get someone to give you a hand to lift a turkey out of the oven. If you have a microwave that is waist high or higher, try using that more often.

Colonial Garden Kitchens, Hanover, PA 17333-0066 Call toll-free 1-800-752-5552 for a free catalog. Mostly household items that are hard to find: like the microwave/TV/utility shelf, a wood chair that's a step stool, a light weight vacuum, full-length body pillows, a wall mount for a TV with a VCR mount below it, appliance rollers, a two-step step stool that folds up thin, telescoping 7½ foot high feather duster, long handled dust pan and broom, wheeled grocery cart, all kinds of space saving racks, a wheeled serving cart.

Comfortably Yours, 2515 East 43rd Street, PO Box 182216, Chattanooga, TN 37422-7216 Call toll free for a catalog 1-800-521-5318 A catalog devoted to your comfort: convoluted foam in three kinds (of which "egg-crate" foam is just one), many pillows, wedges, lap tables, foam cushions for chairs, shower chair, folding canes, portable raised toilet seat, grip bars for the shower, hospital table, foldaway recliner, footstool, 48" long handled sponge for cleaning showers, a heated back cushion for your car or home, expandable bag on wheels, long strapped back scrubber, extending mirror, acupressure insoles, and many other comfort products.

The Selfcare Catalog, 349 Healdsburg Ave., Healdsburg, CA 95448. Call toll free 1-800-345-4021 for a catalog. Started 15 years ago as a magazine called, Medical SelfCare: Access to Medical Tools, this catalog has expanded to health tips, books, videos and equipment: back cushions, yoga, stretching, massage and t'ai chi video, exercise mat, travel pillows, back pad heat massager, strong luggage carrier, cold or hot therapy in pack, ergonomic chairs for home and office, keyboard wrist support, desktop slant, seat wedge, foot massager, pillows, wedges, convoluted foam mattress pad, inversion machine, massage tools, heat massager, insoles, massage tables. Certainly a beautiful catalog.

❍ HEALTH CARE PROVIDER SPECIFIC

Krames Communications, 1100 Grundy Lane, San Bruno, CA 94066-3030, Call 1-800-333-3032. There are a number of

§ *Reduce stress to reduce muscle tension.*

excellent easy-to-read pamphlets published by Krames Communicaations (you may have seen some in your doctors office). Ask for them at your doctor or health care provider's office. Although most of their pamphlets are .40-$2.00 each there is a minimum order of $50.00). As long as you are willing to meet their minimum, anyone can purchase these.

Titles include: Back to Basics, Back Pain, Back Owner's Manual, Back Tips for People Who Sit, Spinal Care, Spinal Degeneration, The Chiropractic Back, Repetitive Strain, Scoliosis, Osteoarthritis, Osteoporosis, Back Pain during Pregnancy and many more. They also sell health and safety materials for the industrial setting which include videos, workbooks *etc.*

Spinal Rehab Supply Co., Inc. 10529C Lakeview Ave, S.W., Tacoma, Wa 98499. Call toll free inside WA state: 1-800-527-3922; outside WA state: 1-800-323-5850. For the professional chiropractor or health care provider: back cushions, wedges, exercise wedges, home traction units, worksheets, models of the spine.

The Saunders Group, 7750 West 78th Street, Bloomington, MN 55439. Call for their corporate oriented catalog of Saunders Therapy Products, toll free 1-800-654-8357

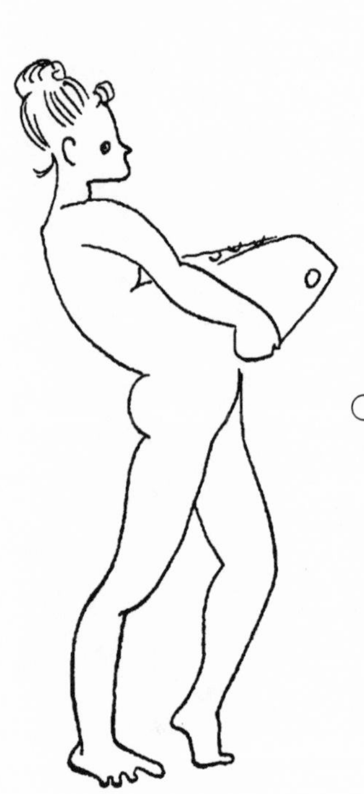

○ CORPORATE BACK PROGRAMS

These groups specialize in bringing the back school to the worker. The emphasis of all of these programs is on prevention. Some have people in the field that can come to your company and train your workers, tailoring a program to your company's individual needs. Others put on seminars across the country where representatives of your company can learn how to put on seminars for your workers. The materials may be a pre-packaged set of videos, workbooks, computer programs, exercise programs or a combination of these materials aimed at low back and/or neck problems, or the materials can be created to meet the needs of your company. It pays to shop around and find out what's available and who can best meet the specific needs of your company. I was quite impressed by the materials of the Saunders Group and ordered some for my own use.

The Back Care Program, author H. Duane Saunders, PT, MS, The Saunders Group, Inc., 7750 W. 78th St., Minneapolis, MN

55439 1-800-654-8357; in MN: 612-944-1656. Contact: H. Duane Saunders.
(This is the most complete and deluxe of these 6 programs).

Back and Neck Care: How to Develop Your Re-education and Prevention Programs, Authors: Stanley V. Paris, PhD, PT and Ronald W , Porter, PT; Vendor: Back School of Atlanta, 1465 Northside Dr., Suite 217, Atlanta, GA 30318, 1-800-783-7536; in GA: 404-355-7756. Contact: Ronald W. Porter

Back at Work, Authors: Don R. Powell, PhD, and Carole Singer, MEd; Vendor: American Institute for Preventive Medicine, 24450 Evergreen, Southfield, MI 48075, 1-800-345-AIPM. In Michigan: 313-352-7666. contact: Don R. Powell

Back Power, Author: David Imrie, MD; Vendor: National Safety Council, 1121 Spring Lake Dr., Itasca, IL 60143-3201, 1-800-621-7619; in IL: 708-285-1121.Contact: Gary Fisher

Corporate Back Safety. Author: David W. Apts, PT; Vendor: American Back School, 5936 Swanson Dr., Ashland, KY 41105-1193, 1-800-637-BACK; in KY: 606-329-9101.Contact: Gene Daniel

How to Protect Your Back. Authors: Hamilton Hall, MD, Maureen Hunt, PT, and Paul Terry, MPH, PhD; Vendor: Staywell Health Management Systems Inc., 1285 Corporate Center Dr., Suite 100, Eagan, MN 55121, 612-454-3577. Contact: David Anderson

Industrial Back Injury Prevention Program. Authors: Nancy Selby, Beth Melton, Cathy Mixson; Vendor: Spine Education Center, Inc. 616 Harry Hines, Suite 302, Dallas TX 75235, 1-800-257-1485; in TX: 214-631-3599.

Industrial Personal Protective Equipment and Programs. Ergodyne Corporation, 1410 Energy Park Dr., Suite 1, St. Paul, MN 55108, 1-800-225-8238; in MN: 612-642-9889.

§ *Avoid lifting. Use handcarts, dollies or other devices to aid in moving and lifting materials. Handcarts and hoists are real bargains, especially compared to hospital fees.*

❍ BACK SCHOOLS

These are back schools at a specific location where the patient can recieve hands-on help. Most often these back schools require a prescription from a doctor for physical therapy. If none of these back schools are near you, call the closest one and ask if they know of one in your area. The following list is by no means complete, nor is it meant to recommend one program over the other. These are just

§ *Under no conditions should you consider using a pushmower. Push mowing and snow shoveling are jobs better left to someone else.*

some of the more well known programs that have a track record for getting the back pain patients back on their feet.

In random calls to back schools across America (using the yellow pages-often listed under physical therapists), there was a wide disparity of types of programs and duration of the program. There are no national guidelines for what constitutes a back school program. There is also no national standardization for back schools. Please check out the section on Back Schools in this book to refamiliarize yourself with what constitutes a good back school program. If you live close to one of these programs, you may want to start here.

California

- *SpineCare Medical Group, Daly City(offices in Portola Valley, Sunnyvale, Fremont, Oakland, and Walnut Creek)*
- *Spine Center of the East Bay, Oakland*
- *St. Mary's Spine Center, San Francisco*
- *San Francisco Spine Center, Saint Francis Memorial Hospital, San Francisco*

Florida

- *St. Francis Hospital Spine Center and Back School, Miami Beach*
- *University of Miami School of Medicine, Pain and Low Back Rehabilitation Program, Miami,*

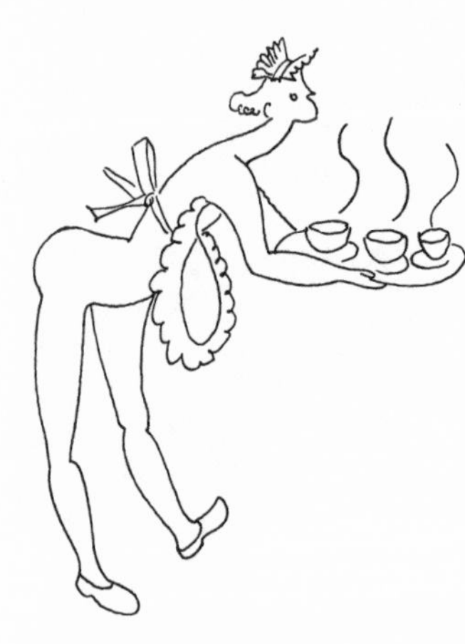

Georgia

- *Atlanta Back School, Atlanta*

Kentucky

- *American Back School, Ashland*

Massachusetts

- *Vanderbilt University, Department of Orthopedics and Rehabilitation, Boston*

Maryland

- *Bethesda Healing Arts Center, Inc. (formerly the Bethesda Back School), Bethesda*

Minnesota

- *Institute of Low Back Care, Minneapolis*
- *Mayo Clinic's Back Center, Rochester*

Pennsylvania

- *PA Back In Action Program Presbyterian-University of Pennsylvania Hospital, Philadelphia*

Tennessee

- *Knoxville Back Care Center, Knoxville, TN*

Texas

- *Texas Back Institute, Dallas, Midland/Odessa, Plano, Houston*
- *Dallas Spinal Rehabilitation Center, Inc., Dallas*

Canada

- *Canadian Back Institute, in operation since 1974, now includes 14 clinics across Canada. These centers are linked by computer. They take a "low-tech" approach to back care and generated a 93% return to work rate with only a 3% reoccurrence of back injury.*

§ *Get a bath brush for washing your back or a loofah with long straps to hold, or a long nylon back scrubber so you don't have to twist and reach just to wash your back.*

❍ HOSPITALS

This list is not meant to be taken as a recommendation for any one hospital. These are just some of the hospitals known for their back surgery. The American Medical Association recommends that you contact the largest hospital in one of the largest cities near you and see if they know of a hospital in your state that specializes in orthopedics (especially as it relates to your specific problem *i.e.* low backs or necks). It is often the case that a doctor, or group of doctors, who specialize in back pain and surgery become well known for their talents. However, if they leave that hospital to open their own private practice, or to associate with another hospital, the emphasis of specialization may change or the quality of the program may be affected.

Please take the time to go back and read the section on SURGERY one more time. This might help you to know what to look for when deciding on a hospital. If there is a good back school in your area, chances are good that they are associated with a hospital. The advantage is that you can get pre- and post-operative help in rehabilitation, or the back school program may eliminate the need for surgery altogether. Texas Back Institute, which is affiliated with three hospitals but refers less than 10% of their patients to surgery, has a free back pain hotline, 1-800-247-BACK. You might want to give them a call first.

California

- ◇ *St. Francis Hospital, San Francisco*
- ◇ *St. Mary's Hospital and Medical Center, St. Mary's Spine Center, San Francisco*
- ◇ *San Francisco Spine Institute at Seton Medical Center, Daly City*
- ◇ *University of California at Irvine, Irvine*
- ◇ **UCLA-University of California at Los Angeles, Los Angeles*
- ◇ *University of California at San Diego, San Diego*

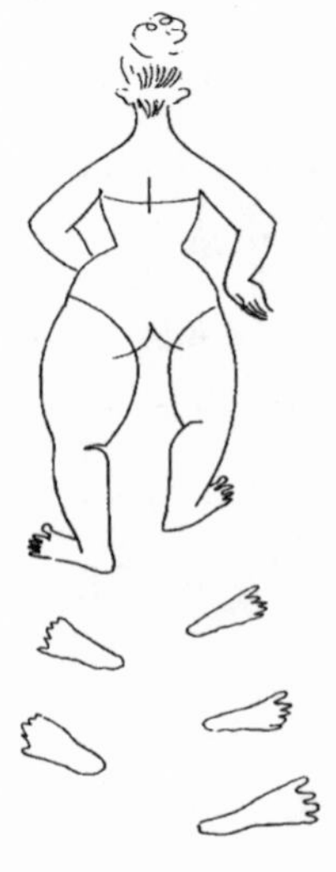

District of Columbia

- ◇ *Georgetown University, Washington*

Florida

- ◇ *St. Francis Hospital Spine Center and Back School, Miami*
- ◇ *University of Miami School of Medicine, Miami*

Iowa

- ◇ *University of Iowa Hospitals and Clinics, Iowa City*

Illinois

- ◇ *Rush-Presbyterian-St. Luke's Medical Center, Chicago*

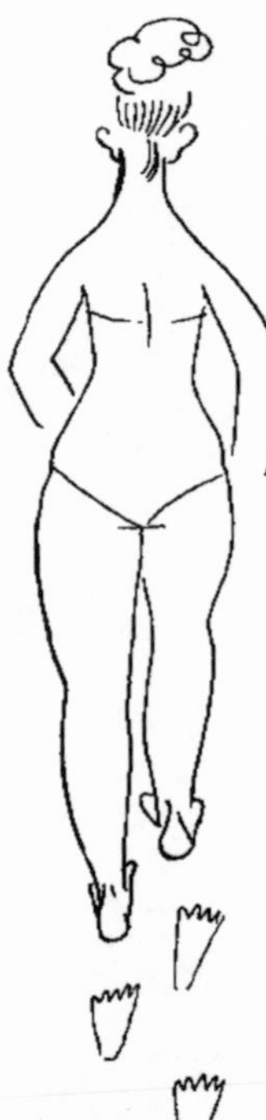

Massachusetts

- ◇ **Brigham and Women's Hospital, Boston*
- ◇ **Massachusetts General Hospital, Boston*

Maryland

- ◇ *Johns Hopkins Hospital, Baltimore*

Minnesota

- ◇ **Mayo Clinic, Rochester*

Missouri

- ◇ *Charles E. Still Osteopathic Hospital, Jefferson City*

New York

- ◇ **Hospital for Special Surgery, New York*
- ◇ *New York University Medical Center, New York City*
- ◇ *Orthopaedic Institute of New York City, New York City*

Oregon

- ◇ *Oregon Health Sciences University Hospital, Portland*

Tennessee

- *Vanderbilt University School of Medicine, Nashville*

Texas

- *Texas Back Institute Affiliates*
- *HCA Medical Center of Plano, Plano*
- *Medical City Hospital, Dallas*
- *St. Joseph's Hospital, Houston*
- *Dallas Specialty Hospital, Dallas*

Vermont

- *University of Vermont College of Medicine, Burlington*

West Virginia

- *Marshall University Medical School, Morgantown*

---

*Rated the top hospitals in America for general othopedics, in a survey of 965 doctors by U.S. News and World Report, 5 August 1991.

§ *Make sure your bed is solid, not sagging. You need not sleep on a hard bed, but chances are that sleeping on a sagging or "rutted" bed will leave you sore all over. If you use box springs, make sure they are firm.*

❍ PAIN CLINICS

These are just a few of the hundreds of pain clinics in America. If you have gotten no relief from doctors or back schools, and it has been four to six months since the onset of pain, these clinics may provide you with the help you need. To get an expert opinion, call the rehabilitation or pain program of your local university medical school.

Long-term chronic pain can not be relieved overnight. It takes time to recondition the body and the mind to overcome pain. Here are some questions you might want to ask before deciding on a pain clinic:

- *How long is your program and how much does it cost?*
- *What is the rate of return to work?*
- *Who oversees this program? (It should be either a specialist in rehabilitative medicine, a medical professional, or your own general practioner).*
- *What happens if this doesn't work? surgery? more rehabilitation programs? Who decides?*
- *Is this an on-going program, or can I set specific goals to accomplish while I am in the program? How can I achieve the highest possible level of activity given my present situation?*

§ *A raised toilet seat helps enormously if you are having or have had surgery or are in great pain. Most people have no idea how low toilet seats really are until they have back problems.*

Arizona

- *Arizona Pain Clinic, Tuscon, Arizona*

California

- *University of California San Francisco Pain Clinic, San Francisco*
- *University of California Los Angeles Pain Management Center, Los Angeles*

Colorado

- *Boulder Memorial Hospital Pain Rehabilitation Program, Boulder*

Connectict

- *Yale Center for Pain Management, New Haven*

District of Columbia

- *Georgetown University Hospital Pain Clinic, Washington*

Florida

- *University of Miami Comprehensive Pain and Rehabilitation Center at Miami Beach's South Shore Hospital, Miami*

Illinois

- *University of Illinois Hospital, Chicago*

Massachusetts

- *Beth Israel Hospital Pain Management Center, Boston*
- *University of Massachusetts Medical Center – Pain Control Center, Worchester*

Michigan

- *Universtiy of Michigan – Coordinated Chronic Pain Program, Ann Arbor*

Minnesota

- **Mayo Clinic – Pain Clinic and Pain Management Center, Rochester*

Missouri

- *Charles E. Still Hospital – Jefferson City Rehabilitation Center, Jefferson City*

Nebraska

- *University of Nebraska Medical Center / Pain Management Center, Omaha*

New Jersey

- *University of Medicine and Dentistry-New Jersey Medical School Pain Management Center, Newark*

§ *Don't sit if you can stand, don't stand if you can lay down, is sage advice.*

New York

- *Columbia – Presbyterian Medical Center Pain Treatment Service, New York*
- *New York University Medical Center Comprehensive Pain Center, New York*
- *Orthopaedic-Arthritis Pain Center, New York*
- **Rusk Institute of Rehabilitation Medicine, New York*

Ohio

- *Ohio State University Chronic Pain Program, Columbus*

Pennsylvania

- *University of Pittsburgh Center for Pain Evaluation and Treatment, Pittsburgh*

Tennessee

- *Vanderbilt University Medical Center Ability Assessment Center, Nashville, TN and Vanderbilt Pain Control Center, Nashville*

Texas

- *Dallas Spinal Rehabilitation Center, Inc., Spinal and Chronic Pain Program, Dallas*
- *University of Texas Center for Pain Medicine at Herman, Houston*

Washington

- **University of Washington Medical Center, Multidisciplinary Pain Center, Seattle, WA*

* Rated among the top seven general rehabilitation hospitals in America, in a survey by U.S. News & World Report, August 5, 1991.

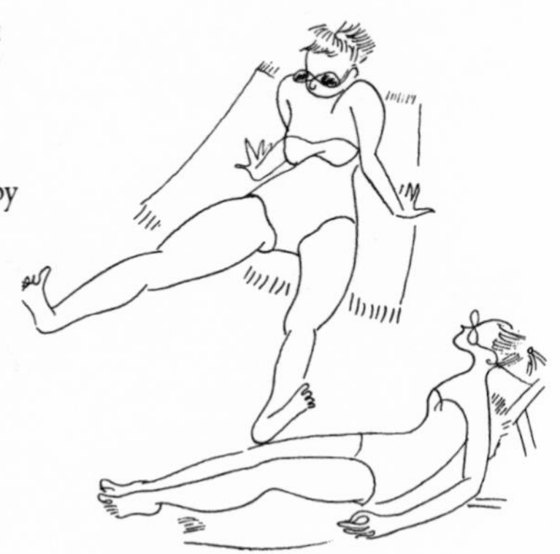

SUGGESTED READING LIST

Abraham, Edward A., MD. Freedom from Back Pain. Emmaus, PA: Rodale Press, 1986.

American Medical Association Guide to Backcare. New York: Random House, 1984.

Bove, Alexander. *Medicaid Planning Handbook.* Boston: Little, Brown, 1992.

Donkin, Scott W., DC. *Sitting on the Job: How to Survive the Stresses of Sitting Down to Work – A Practical Handbook.* Boston: Houghton Mifflin Company, 1989.

Gach, Michael Reed. *The Bum Back Book: Acupressure Self Help Back Care for Relieving Pain and Tension.* Berkeley, CA: Celestial Arts, 1983.

Hall, Hamilton, MD. *The Back Doctor.* New York: Berkeley Books, 1982.

Klein, Arthur C., and Dava Sobel. *Backache Relief.* New York: Signet NAL, 1986.

Lettvin, Maggie. *Maggie's Back Book.* Boston: Houghton Mifflin Company, 1976.

Maddox, Sam. *Spinal Network: The Total Resource for the Wheelchair Community.* Boulder, CO: Spinal Network, 1990.

McKenzie, Robin. *Treat Your Own Back.* Waikanae, New Zealand: Spinal Publications Ltd., 1985

McKenzie, Robin. *Treat Your Own Neck.* Waikanae, New Zealand: Spinal Publications Ltd., 1983.

Melleby, Alexander. *The Y's Way to a Healthy Back.* New Jersey: New Century Publishers, Inc., 1982.

Perlroth, Karen A., and Ellen Lagerwerff. *Mensendieck, Your Posture: Encountering Gravity the Correct and Beautiful Way.* Chicago: Aries Press, 1982.

Root, Leon, MD and Thomas Kiernan. *Oh, My Aching Back.* New York: Signet NAL, 1985.

Schuler, Stephen Hosck, MD. *Back in Shape.* Boston: Houghton Mifflin Company, 1991.

White, Augustus A. III, MD. *Your Aching Back.* New York: Simon & Schuster (Fireside), 1990.

§ *Vacuuming, raking leaves and sweeping all require that you "walk your tool" — walk with your vacuum, pull the rake and sweep with short, even motions. Or use a lunging motion, where you move from your hips, not your back.*

❍ FOR MORE INFORMATION

On Specific Doctors in Your Area

American Academy of Family Physicians

8880 Ward Parkway
Kansas City, MO 64114
(800) 274-2237
A national association of family doctors.

American Academy of Physical Medicine and Rehabilitation

122 S. Michigan Ave., Suite 1300
Chicago, IL 60603
Write for a list of physiatrists in your area.

§ *If you watch TV in bed, put it up high. There are shelves and mounting fixtures available. This way you don't have to contort your body just to watch the evening program.*

For help in finding a qualified chiropractor in your area or if you have questions on chiropractic care

American Chiropractic Association

1701 Clarendon Blvd.
Arlington, VA 22209
(800) 368-3083

American Osteopathic Association

142 East Ontario
Chicago, IL 60611
(800) 621-1773
Offers information and local referrals on osteopathic medicine

North American Spine Association

222 S. Prospect Ave. #127
Park Ridge, IL 60068
(708) 698-1628
They offer names of orthopedic spine surgeons, radiologists and neurosurgeons in your area, but not referrals

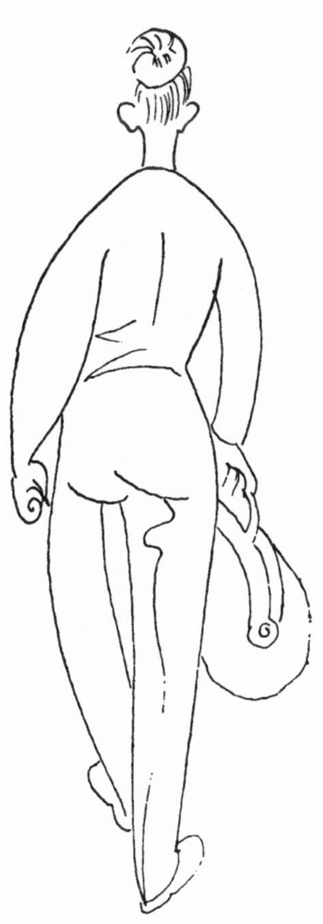

❍ ON BODYWORK AND BODYWORKERS

American Massage Therapy Association

1130 W. North Shore Ave.
Chicago, IL 60626
(312) 761-AMTA
They offer referrals to a variety of qualified bodyworkers through state chapters. Call or write for free information packet on massage in America.

North American Society of Teachers of the Alexander Technique (NASTAT)

PO Box 3992
Champaign, IL 61826
(217) 359-3529

Call or write for free information packet, including a national list of certified instructors.

❍ ON BACK PAIN

Texas Back Institute

Back Pain Hotline
(800) 247-Back (Toll free)
A hotline for those in pain from back trouble.

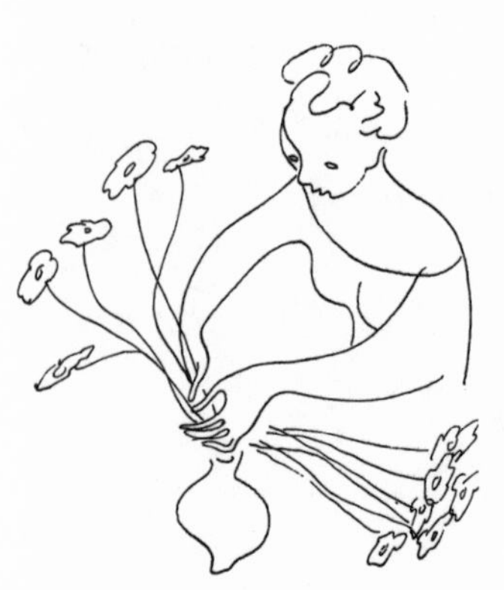

American Academy of Orthopaedic Surgeons
222 South Prospect Ave.
Park Ridge, Il 60068-4058
(708) 823-7186

They publish a pamphlet on low back pain. Single copies are available free with a #10 (legal size) self-addressed envelope to:
PO Box 618
Park Ridge, IL 60068

❍ ON PAIN

American Chronic Pain Association, Inc.

PO Box 850
Rocklin, CA 95677
(916) 632-0922

National Chronic Pain Outreach Association

7979 Old Georgetown Rd.
Suite 100
Bethesda, MD 20814-2429
(301) 652-4948

❍ ON COMPREHENSIVE HEALTH ISSUES

ODPHD National Health Information Center

PO Box 1133
Washington, D.C. 20013
(800) 336-4797

Provides information and referrals for consumers interested in a wide variety of health information.

§ Wear shoes that don't lace up.

National Organization for Rare Disorders (NORD)

PO Box 8923
New Fairfield, CT 06812
(203) 746-6518
(800) 447-6673 (Toll free)

National Institute of Arthritis and Musculoskeletal and Skin Diseases

Office of Scientific and Health Communications
Building 31, Room 4C05
Bethesda, MD 20892
(301) 496-8188

National Institute of Neurological Disorders and Stroke

Department of Health and Human Services
Public Health Service – National Institutes of Health
Bldg. 31 Room 8A06
Bethesda, MD 20892
(301) 496-5751

Ask for their 27 page pamphlet on Chronic Pain and their back pain fact sheet.

❍ ON ARTHRITIS

Arthritis Foundation

1314 Spring St. N.W.
Atlanta, GA 30309
(404) 872-7100
(800) 283-7800 (Toll free)

They publish quite a few pamphlets on arthritis. They can also refer you to an area chapter closer to you.

Arthritis Consulting Services

4620 North State Rd. 7
Suite 206
Ft. Lauderdale, FL 33319
(800) 327-3027 (Toll free)

Provides answers to questions about arthritis and a free booklet.

§ *Get a telephone near your bed. Surround yourself with all the things you might need before you get in bed (tissues, books, water, paper, pen. . .)*

❍ ON HEAD INJURY

National Head Injury Foundation

1140 Connecticut Ave., NW
Suite 812
Washington, DC 20036
(202) 296-6443
(800) 444-NIHF (Toll Free)

❍ ON REHABILITATION

National Rehabilitation Information Center (NARIC)

Macro Systems-Suite 935
8455 Colesville Rd.
Silver Springs, MD 20910-3319
(301) 588-9284
(800) 364-2742 (Toll Free)

National Institute on Disability and Rehabilitation Research (NIDRR)

Department of Education
330 C St., S.W., Room 3060
Washington, DC 20202-2572
(202) 732-1134

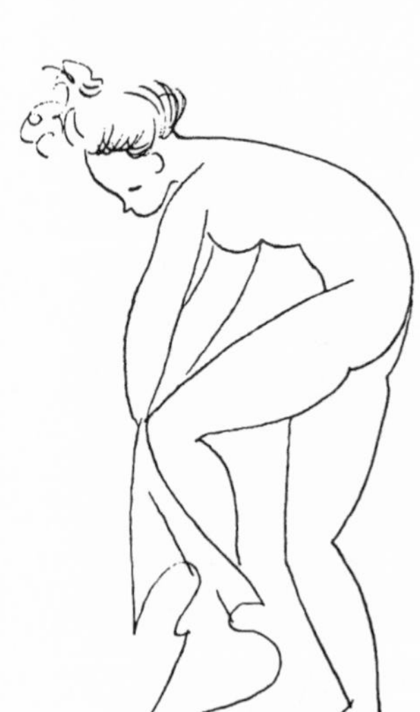

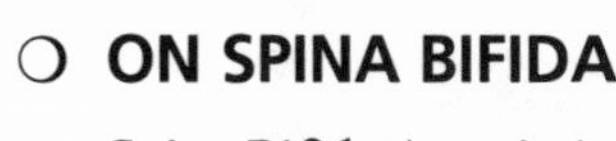

❍ ON SPINA BIFIDA

Spina Bifida Association of America

1700 Rockville Pike, Suite 540
Rockville, MD 20852
(301) 770-SBAA (7222)
(800) 621-3141 (Toll free)

❍ ON SPINAL CHORD INJURIES

National Spinal Cord Injury Association

600 West Cummings Park, Suite 600
Woburn, MA 01801
(800) 962-9629

An invaluable resource is the book *Spinal Network: The Total Resource for the Wheelchair Community*. Nationwide support groups provide information on spinal cord injury, prevention and research. Phone: 1-800-338-5412.

ON SPINAL MUSCULAR ATROPHY

Families of Spinal Muscular Atrophy

PO Box 1465
Highland Park, IL 60035
(708) 432-5551

ON TUBEROUS SCLEROSIS

National Tuberous Sclerosis Association

8000 Corporate Dr., Suite 120
Landover, MD 20785
(301) 459-9888
(800) 225-6872 (Toll free)

SOURCES

Abraham, Edward. *Freedom From Back Pain.* Rodale Press, 1986

Alper, Joseph. "Back Pain." Washington Post Health. 11 July 1989. *Annals of Internal Medicine,* v. 112, no.8, April 15, 1990.

Arthritis Foundation. *Primer on the Rheumatic Diseases,* Ninth Edition. 1988.

Back Tips for Health Care Providers. Daly City, CA: Krames Communications, 1986.

Borenstein, David. "Low back pain: epidemiology, etiology, diagnostic evaluation, and therapy." *Current Science.* 1991

Borenstein, David G., MD and Sam W. Weisel, MD. *Low Back Pain: Medical Diagnosis and Comprehensive Management.* Philadelphia: WB Saunders Company, 1989.

Boyd, Brendan. *San Francisco Chronicle,* 23 August 1991.

Brodsky, Ruthan. "How to play a good game with a bad back." New Choices. April 1991.

Changing Times. "Back Workouts That Work." June 1988.

§ *Use a long-handled shoe horn.*

Fast, Abital, MD. "Low Back Disorders: Conservative Management." *Archives of Physical Medicine and Rehabilitation,* Vol 69, October 1988

Ferm, Vergilius. *A Brief Dictionary of American Superstitions,* New York: Philosophical Library, 1959.

Folklore Archives. University of California, Berkeley, CA: Superstitions, Folkspeech, Folkspeech Cautionary.

Frymoyer, John, MD. "Low back pain: Medicine's most challenging symptom." *PA Practice* 4(3). 1985.

Glamour. "8 Ways to Prevent Back Pain." Beauty and Health Report. Vol. 87 (Feb. 89).

Grossman, Richard M. Cited by Joseph Alper. "Back Pain," *Washington Post Health.* 11 July 1989.

Jackson, Mildred. *The Handbook of Alternatives to Chemical Medicine,* Oakland, CA: Lawton-Teague Publications, 1975.

Kirkaldy-Willis, William H., MA, MD, FRCS, FACS. *Managing Low Back Pain.* New York: Churchill Livingstone, 1988.

Klein, Arthur C., and Dava Sobel. *Backache Relief.* New York: Times Books (Random House), 1988.

Leary, Warren E. Quoting Dr. Javid. "Drug Is Given New Chance as Cure for Back Pain," *The New York Times*, 13 July 1989.

McCloy, Marjorie and Sophie Taggart. "Back In Action." *Woman's Sports and Fitness* 12, Sept. 1990.

Meyer, Clarence. *Vegetarian Medicines.* Glenwood, IL: Meyer Books, 1981.

Mills, Simon, M.A. *Alternatives in Healing.* New American Library, 1988.

Pearson, Ridley. "Hindsight." Back In Action, *AIMPLUS.* April 1988.

Pedinoff, Seymour, DO et al. "Motion and Progress in Low-Back Pain." *Patient Care.* 15 May 1991.

Prevention Magazine. "Put an End to Backaches." Aug. 1988.

Robert, Rickard. "Yoga For Your Back," *Men's Health,* Winter 1988.

Rose, Jeanne. *Herbs and Things: Jeanne Rose's Herbal,* New York: Grosset & Dunlap, 1972.

Southmayd, William, *MD. Sports Health: The Complete Book of Athletic Injuries.* Quick Fox, 1981.

Stevenson, Burton. *The Home Book of Quotations: Classical and Modern.* New York: Dodd, Mead and Company, 1967.

Tevis, Cheryl. "Staying on Top of 'Tractor Back'." *Successful Farming,* March 1990.

Thesen, Karen. *Country Remedies from Pantry, Field and Garden.* London: Harper Colophon Books, 1979.

United States Department of Health and Human Services. *Report on Low Back Pain.* Nov. 1987.

USA Today. "Can You Avoid Aches and Pain?" Vol. 118 (Oct. 89). *U.S. News and World Report,* 5 August 1991: 61.

White, Arthur. "Back In Action." *Shape.* June 1991.

White, Augustus A. III, MD. *Your Aching Back: A Doctor's Guide to Relief,* revised ed. New York: Fireside (Simon & Schuster), 1990.

Wyngaarden, James B. MD, and Lloyd H. Smith, Jr. MD, Eds. Cecil *Textbook of Medicine, 18th Edition.* Philadelphia, PA: W.B. Saunders Company (Harcourt Brace Jovanovich), 1988.

§ *Use the inexpensive device made for helping to put on socks.*

DOS, DON'TS, QUOTES, etc.

Don't lunge to catch falling objects. This is a sure way to throw your back out of whack.

Don't lift anything from the floor without getting close to the object and then getting down on one knee.

Don't overdo it! When you're rushed, stressed out, tired or panicked, your back is set up for a strain.

Don't just sit around—we go from sitting at the breakfast table to sitting in our car, to sitting at work, to sitting in the car. And then we get home and have to sit down because we're so tired (basically from sitting). Then we sit to eat, watch TV or read in bed.

Don't bend from the waist to lift anything, or reach for something on the floor.

Don't stand without resting one foot on a stepstool. This takes pressure off the lower back and discs.

Don't lean over to brush your teeth, shave, put on makeup. Stand with one foot in front of the other and bend from the hips, not the waist.

Don't bend at the waist.

Don't lift and twist at the same time.

Don't lay on your stomach.

Don't hold the phone between your head and shoulder.

Don't jump out of bed, a chair, or jump up off the floor unless the house is burning.

Don't lay on your side with your elbow bent and your hand holding your head. You're twisting your head, neck and lower back.

§ *Invest in a lot of throw pillows so you can put one or two on your lap when you read. By bringing the reading surface up to your eyes you avoid straining your neck or back.*

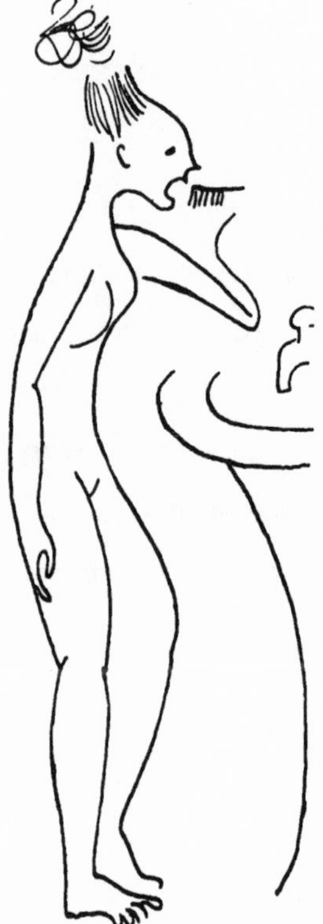

Don't jump up and down to reach a short pull cord or something on a shelf. This puts enormous pressure on your discs.
Don't lift a heavy object higher than your waist.
Don't carry unbalanced loads.
Don't overload your purse, pack or arms.
Don't lift or move heavy furniture.
Don't sit in soft chairs.
Don't change from high heel to flats. Wear moderate heels.
Don't stoop and stretch to hang wash, bring the clothes basket higher and the clothes line lower.
Don't slouch.
Don't strain to open windows or doors.
Don't bend over to pick up children's toys. Get them to do it. Or, get down on your knees before scooping them up.
Don't bend over to pick an infant or small child up off the floor. Always get down on one knee first.
Don't bend over from the waist to get an infant or small child out of a stroller. Bend your knees keeping your back straight and lift with your legs (this is a great thigh workout).
Don't bend and twist to get a child out of a car seat in the back of a two-door car. Put the child up front, or think about a four-door car.
Don't bend your neck and shoulders to read a book in your lap or flat on a desk. Bring the book up to your eyes by either putting two pillows on your lap first, using a slantboard on a desk, propping the book up on top of other books or by putting your elbows on the desk to hold the book at eye level. In the kitchen, cookbooks can be put in a plastic cookbook holder. For typing or computer work use a copy holder, or your cookbook holder on top of a box.
Don't carry grocery bags that are too heavy. Better to make more trips with lighter bags.
Don't bend over to put on socks, shoes, pants or other clothing. Sit down!
Don't get into a car without first putting down whatever is in your arms.
Don't buy clothes that button up the back unless someone else can button them up for you.
Don't bend over wash tub sinks that are very deep. Two plastic coated dish drainers (of different sizes) turned upside down

and stacked perpendicular to each other will bring the bottom of the sink up to you. Then a plastic tub can be put on top of that. (This will take some experimenting as dish drainers and sinks tend to differ in size).

❍ FOLKLORE

§ *Be sure your equipment has tongue jacks. Hitching to an implement in a hurry is one way to spend two weeks staring at the ceiling.*

Step on a crack, you break your mother's back.
Step on a line, break your mother's spine.
It may be some kind of homeopathic magic which might be under the control of the individual.
– Folklore Archives-U. of CA, Berkeley, CA, Superstitions II D5A25

Don't bend so low that your derrier won't go.
Don't try to do anything beyond your capabilities.
– circa 1915. Folklore Archives-U. of CA, Berkeley, CA, Folkspeech, VI c3

Make your head save your heels.
You can create less work and wear and tear on yourself if you think ahead.
– Folklore Archives-U. of CA, Berkeley, CA, Folkspeech VI c3

E. Texas (references to Scotland, Western U.S.)

Don't get your back up.
"Don't get angry." Reference to animals when they get upset and ready to fight.
– Folklore Archives-U. of CA, Berkeley, CA, Folkspeech Cautionary VI c3

Wahington Cascades by N. Carolinians

Don't rush away in the heat of the day without your blankets.
It may be hot now, but plan for later.
– Folklore Archives-U. of CA, Berkeley, CA, Folkspeech VI c3

Lake Co.

You can see the mortician from the hospital.
"Don't go to the big city hospital because if you do you'll die."
Instead of having family around, the mortician would be waiting for business.
– Folklore Archives-U. of CA, Berkeley, CA, Folkspeech VI c3 1974

He's on my back.
To describe someone who is hassling you, or giving you a bad time.
– Folklore Archives-U. of CA, Berkeley, CA, Folkspeech (Occupational Medicine, Dental) XVIM4

§ *Vacuuming, raking leaves and sweeping all require that you "walk your tool"— walk with your vacuum, pull the rake and sweep with short, even motions. Or use a lunging motion, where you move from your hips, not your back.*

You're hurtin' for certain.
Looking for trouble (much like the phrase "cruisin' for a bruisin).
zapper-x-rays

❍ FOLK MEDICINE

Oklahoma

For aches and pains, mix a tablespoon of vinegar and honey together, and then drink the mixture. For arthritis and rheumatism – also good for aches in the bones; "It will grease the joints."

– Folklore Archives U. of CA, Superstitions II D5 A25

Cure for Backache: "*Have a 2 year old child urinate on your back.*"
Folklore Archive- U. of CA, Berkeley, CA, Superstitions II D5 A25

Switzerland, 1894

Put a potato in your pocket and keep it there to cure pain.
If it shrinks and turns to stone, keep it there so the pain won't come back. If the pain is not stopped by the time the potato is dried, put a new one in your pocket.

– Folklore Archives- U. of CA, Berkeley, CA Superstitions II D5A25

Minnesota, 1905

A poultice used for sore and inflamed parts of the body is a mustard plaster. Mustard plasters are made with dry mustard and hot water and are laid upon the inflamed region to supposedly draw out pain. They are left on for only a short time, for if they dry they are painful to remove.

– Folklore Archives-U. of CA, Berkeley, CA, Superstition II-D5A25

New England:

Peel a potatoe carry it in your pocket: this is good for rheumatism.

– Vergilius Ferm, *A Brief Dictionary of American Superstitions,* New York: Philosophical Library, 1959.

Maine:

Buckshot carried in the hip pocket will prevent rheumatism; turtle shell ashes will cure it.

– Vergilius Ferm, *A Brief Dictionary of American Superstitions,* New York: Philosophical Library, 1959.

Sciatica may be relieved by the use of a plaster of onions, rum and neet's foot-oil on the hip.

– Vergilius Ferm, *A Brief Dictionary of American Superstitions*, New York: Philosophical Library, 1959.

Sleeping on a bearskin rug will cure a backache.

– Vergilius Ferm, *A Brief Dictionary of American Superstitions*, New York: Philosophical Library, 1959.

Cow manure as a poltice is good for aches and pains.

– Vergilius Ferm, *A Brief Dictionary of American Superstitions*, New York: Philosophical Library, 1959.

§ *Stay away from high heels that increase swayback.*

❍ Cure for Aching Muscles:

Put alcohol into a cup filling it about a third full. Light the alcohol. Flip the cup over onto the spot where the muscles are hurting. The flame goes out, using the air in the cup and creates a vacuum and pulls out the muscles.

– Folklore Archives, U. of CA, Berkeley, CA, Superstitions II-D5A25

One ascorbic acid tablet taken daily prevents backaches. "Patient with ruptured disc tried it and it doesn't work."

– Folklore Archives-U. of CA, Berkeley, CA, Superstitions II D5A25

For sprains you use a grated potato poultice. You grate the potato and let them stand in a strainer until the juice is drained off, then put the grated potato in a cloth and fold it over and put it on the sprain. Sleep with it overnight and in the morning it will be much relieved. Put a plastic bag over the potato cloth if you want to avoid juice in your bed.

– Folklore Archives-U. of CA, Berkeley, CA, Superstitions D5A25

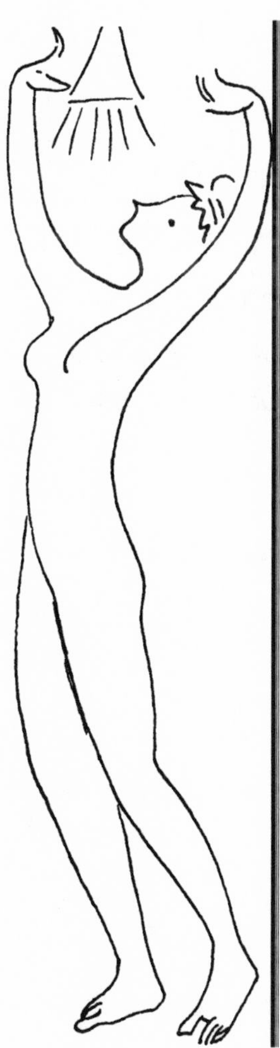

❍ Muscular Pains

A rustic recipe: rub aching parts with slices of raw potato or raw onions.

– Clarence Meyer. Vegetarian Medicines. Glenwood, IL: Meyer Books, 1981.

European peasants make a paste [a mess] with barley bran, barley meal, a little vinegar and butter. The paste is heated and applied warm to painful areas.

– Clarence Meyer. *Vegetarian Medicines*. Glenwood, IL: Meyer Books, 1981.

Sciatica

Germans believe eatring an abundance of raw sauerkraut helps prevent sciatica.

– Clarence Meyer. V*egetarian Medicines*. Glenwood, IL: Meyer Books, 1981.

Minced fresh horseradish root is used like mustard seed as a stimulating poultice applied for neuralgia, sciatica, cramps etc.

– Clarence Meyer. *Vegetarian Medicines*. Glenwood, IL: Meyer Books, 1981.

An old English physician advised celery tea, hot and strong (with cream and sugar, if desired), to be drunk by the teacupful 3 to 4 times in the day, so as to abate neuralgia and sciatica, which it sometimes will do very speedily.

– Clarence Meyer. *Vegetarian Medicines*. Glenwood, IL: Meyer Books, 1981.

Doctor Bartie's Medicine for aches and swellings. I haven't been able to discover just who Dr. Bartie was but he is quoted as an authority in The Good Hus-wives Jewell (1597). 'Take flowers of camomile and rose leaves, steep them in white wine, making a plaister therof, lay it ont the place where any pain, ache or swelling is.'

– Karen Thesen. *Country Remedies from Pantry, Field and Garden*. London: Harper Colophon Books, 1979.

❍ Comfrey Poultice

For thousands of years comfrey has been used to promote healings of wounds, ulcers and fractured bones. This is a soothing poultice which brings great relief to sprains and muscular aches and pains.

- *2 handfuls fresh comfrey leaves*
- *1 pint (2½ cups) boiling water*

Chop the comfrey leaves finely, pour the boiling water over and soak for 5 minutes. Drain, and spread the leaves on to a cloth wrung out in hot water. Fold this over and apply to the affected part. Bind with a dry bandage and renew the poultice as necessary. It is important to use fresh comfrey leaves for each new poultice, not just to reheat the old ones.

– Karen Thesen. *Country Remedies from Pantry, Field and Garden*. London: Harper Colophon Books, 1979.

§ *"Causes of physical impotence in men in the United States due to spinal cord injury is 8%.*

❍ QUOTES

"And a crook in his back,
And a melancholy crack
In his laugh."

– Oliver Wendell Holmes, *The Last Leaf*

Burton Stevenson. The Home Book of Quotations: Classical and Modern, 28:3. New York: Dodd, Mead and Company, 1967.

"The back is made for the burden."

– Thomas Carlyle, quoted as "a pious adage."
Burton Stevenson. *The Home Book of Quotations: Classical and Modern*, 204:12. New York: Dodd, Mead and Company, 1967.

"Pain is forgotten where gain comes."
– John Ray, *English Proverbs*

Burton Stevenson. *The Home Book of Quotations: Classical and Modern,* 1444:18. New York: Dodd, Mead and Company, 1967.

"When pain ends, gain ends too."
– Robert Browning, "A Death in the Desert"

Burton Stevenson. *The Home Book of Quotations: Classical and Modern,* 1444:18. New York: Dodd, Mead and Company, 1967.

§ *Jeans that are too tight can cause muscle and nerve problems.*

"I'll rack thee with old cramps,
Fill all thy bones with aches, make thee roar
That beasts shall tremble at thy din."
– Shakespeare, *The Tempest* I.ii.

The Home Book of Quotations: Classical and Modern, New York: Dodd, Mead and Company, 1967

"Atlas, we read in ancient song,
was so exceeding tall and strong,
He bore the skies upon his back,
Just as the peddler does his pack;
But, as the peddler overpress'd
Unloads upon a stall to rest,
Or, when he canno[?] longer stand,
Desires a friend to lend a hand,
So Atlas, lest the ponderous spheres
Should sink, and fall about his ears,
got Hercules to bear the pile,
that he might sit and rest awhile."
– Jonathan Swift, "Atlas; or, the Minister of State"

The Home Book of Quotations: Classical and Modern, New York: Dodd, Mead and Company, 1967

❍ FAMOUS PEOPLE WITH BACK PROBLEMS

RAMSES II (ruler of Egypt from 1292 to 1225 B.C.) – ankylosing spondylitis. His spine was so stiff and curved that his head was bent forward and he could take only tiny steps-but lived to be 90.

IVAN THE TERRIBLE (Russian Czar Ivan IV) – His pain from an extremely twisted spine supposedly led to his disposition as a tyrannical ruler.

HUNCHBACK OF NOTRE DAME – kyphosis

THOMAS JEFFERSON - developed an acute case of backache when he showed his slaves how to use a plow

JOHN FITZGERALD KENNEDY - wartine injury, wore a back brace during his political life, and spent hours in his rocking chair.

While he was writing his autobiography, Profiles in Courage, he underwent 2 long and difficult surgeries. He was known to take a lot of painkillers for his ongoing pain.

EVERETTE KOOP - worked standing up

CYRUS VANCE

SHAKESPEARE - SCIATICA

ERNEST HEMINGWAY - had a nagging back ache and choose to write standing up

EDMUND MUSKIE

PRINCE CHARLES - fell horseback riding. Prince Charles has regular physiotherapist appointments.

ELIZABETH TAYLOR - like Prince Charles, hurt while horseback riding. Taylor fell during filming of National Velvet in 1945. She has had a series of back operations and pain so great it led to a pain pill addiction. Through the Betty Ford Clinic, she has now overcome that addiction.

§ *Don't carry your wallet in your back pocket. Oftentimes that is just enough to set off the sciatic nerve when sitting.*

JOAN SUTHERLAND

BARBARA STREISAND

PRINCESS DI, CYBILL SHEPARD, IVANNA TRUMP - all started back trouble during pregnancy. Princess Di regularly gets her back cracked by a chiropractor and opts for flat shoes for day-to-day wear. Cybill Shepard married her chiropractor. Ivanna Trump keeps the high heels and gets massages twice weekly.

SPORTS

BALLET - VERONICA TENNANT(former Canadian Ballet Star) - herniated discs. Spent nine weeks in a body cast and full recovery lasted one year.

BASEBALL - RICK BULESON(former Boston Red Sox) - spondylolysis

STEVE CARLTON - back spasms

JOE DIMAGGIO - back trouble later in life kept him out of old timers games.

DENNIS ECKERSLEY ('79 ace starter for the Boston Red Sox) - spinal abnormality
CARELTON FISK (former Boston Red Sox) - spondylolysis
RON GUIDRY (NY Yankee pitcher) missed games
MATT KEOUGH (NY Yankee pitcher)
TONY KUBEK (NY Yankee infielder)
GLEN HOFFMAN (Boston Red Sox's third baseman) - lumbar strain
REGGIE JACKSON
JOHN LALLY (trainer for the Washington Bullets) - spondylolistheses
RUDY MAY (Yankee pitcher)
CHUCK NOLL
PETE ROSE
GEORGE "BOOMER' SCOTT (first baseman of the Boston Red Sox) - spondylolisthesis - 50%
ROBIN YOUNT - Milwaukee Brewers All - Star shortstop.
BASKETBALL - PHIL CHENIER (former Washington Bullet); MITCH KUPCHAK (forward of the Washington Bullets) - chronic problems, surgery twice

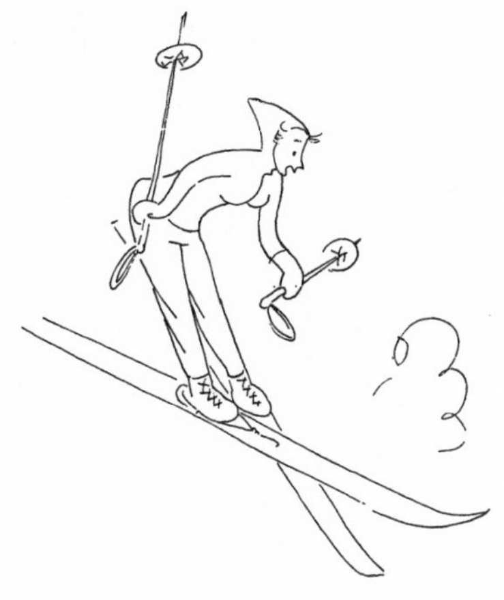

BILL WALTON
LARRY BIRD - back surgery
BOXING - MIKE WEAVER - former heavyweight champion, injury to his lower back.
FOOTBALL - JOE MONTANA - Lower disc problem. Chiropractic manipulation done on TV.
JOE CHARBONEAU - American League rookie of the year 1980, three ruptured discs.
PAT LEAHY - New York Jets punter
TOM SKLADANY (Detroit Lions punter) - ruptured disc removed in the fall of 1979.
GOLF - LEE TREVENO
FUZZY ZOELLER
JACK NICKALAUS - back ailment treated by anatomical functionalist.
GYMNASTICS - OLGA KORBET - 25% spondylolisthesis
ICE HOCKEY - JOHN DAVIDSON - star goalie, injuries to his back
GIL GILBERT - (NY Rangers) back fusion CAMILLE HENRY (NY Rangers) back fusion

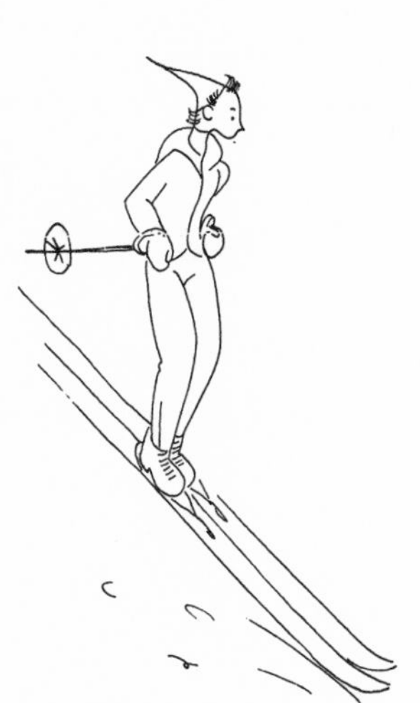

WAYNE GRETZKY (LA Kings) - two injured facet joints, missed 17 games in 1990.
HARRY HOWE (NY RANGERS) back fusion
JEAN RATELLE ('60's high scoring center for Boston Bruins) - herniated disc, back fusion
SKIING - SANDY WILLIAMS (slalom specialist)
SOCCER - WILLINGTON ORTIZ - had surgery for herniated disc; reinjured it later.
TENNIS - TRACY AUSTIN, back pain
BORIS BECKER - chronic back problems
PAT CASH
STEPHAN EDBERG
HANA MANDLIKOVA
JOHN MCENROE
HANA MANDIKOVA
MURISLAV MERCIR

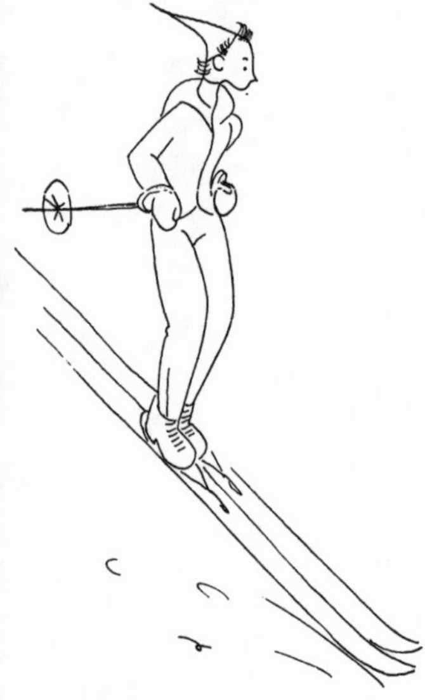

❍ HERBS

from Simon Mills, M.A., *Alternatives in Healing*, New American Library, 1988.

Lime Blossom (Tilia curopea): general relaxant which improves circulation. It helps to reduce tension and insomnia without acting as a sedative.
Cramp Bark (Bivurmon opulus): strong muscle relaxant, acting to reduce both asthmatic spasms and tensions in the skeleton.
Lobelia (lobelia inflata): reduces irritability and inflammation of the airways, helping both sinusitis and asthmatic attacks.
Devil's Claw (Harpagophytun procumbens): analgesic and anti-inflammatory, reducing pain as an aid to long-term balancing of causes.
Valerian (Valerian officinalis): a warming anti-spasmodic, which reduces the muscle tension and calms the nervous system, improving headaches and other symptoms of stress. It relaxes blood vessel walls and improves circulation.

❍ BACK LINES

Back biting
Back against the wall

no backbone
spineless (1827)
have your back up about it
carry. . . on his back
stab in the back/back stabbing/talking behind your back
get off my back
back breaking(1870) extremely tiring or demanding: oppressive
backdown (1849)-to withdraw from a commitment or position
backlog (1684)-a large log at the back of the hearth; an accumulation of unperformed tasks or materials not processed
back off (1954)-back down
back out (1807)-to withdraw from a commitment or contest
back rest (1859) a rest for the back
back seat-inferior position, won't take a . . . to anyone
pain in the neck

INDEX

Colophon

THIS BOOK WAS PRODUCED almost exclusively using MS-DOS desktop publishing facilities. The original manuscript was provided on disk using PC WordPerfect 5.1. Initial coding was done in PC Microsoft Word 5.0. The layout and page make-up was accomplished in Ventura Publisher 4.01a (Windows) on an Orchid 80486-50 local buss system. The majority of the artwork was scanned to .PCX format using a Logitech Scanman and Fototouch. Retouching, where necessary, was done with Micrografx Picture Publisher. Two line drawings were annotated in Corel Draw 2.01L. The aggregate data file size was ~5.4 megabytes. Proofing was accomplished using a QMS 820 Turbo, and final output was produced on a Linotronic 330.

The serif typeface is Monotype Centaur; the sans serif heads are Adobe Frutiger.

– *Fifth Street Design*

SIMPLE CHANGES PACKET

We are pleased to offer a *free* packet of information on *Simple Changes* you can make in your lifestyle (at home, in the office, in your car) that can have a tremendous impact on the way you feel.

To receive your information packet, please fill out this page and send it, along with a Self-Addressed Stamped Envelope, to:

Simple Changes/*The Back Almanac*
P.O. Box 20429
Oakland, CA 94620

You'll be glad you did!

Name ______________________________

Street Address ______________________________

City, State Zip ______________________________

Age: Under 25 ☐ 25-35 ☐ 35-45 ☐ 45-60 ☐ Over 60 ☐

Sex: Male ☐ Female ☐

How often are you bothered by back pain? ______________________________

What do you believe is the problem with your back? ______________________________

____

____

What has been most helpful to you? ______________________________

____

____

Have you ever had back surgery? Yes ☐ *No* ☐ *what kind?* ______________

____

____

What type of over-the-counter treatments/medicines do you use? ______________

____

____

Are you interested in receiving a free catalog of information on helpful products for your back? Yes ☐ No ☐

Would you be interested in providing a brief, written testimonial of your back experience for future editions of the Almanac? Yes ☐ No ☐

OTHER BOOKS FROM *LANIER PUBLISHING*

- *Condo Vacations — The Complete Guide*
- *All-Suite Hotel Guide — The Definitive Directory*
- *Golf Courses — The Complete Guide*
- *Golf Resorts— The Complete Guide*
- *Golf Resorts International*
- *Complete Guide to Bed & Breakfast Inns & Guesthouses*
- *22 days in Alaska*
- *Cinnamon Mornings*
- *Elegant Small Hotels — A Connoisseur's Guide*

For order and further information, please contact:

Lanier Publishing International, Ltd.
Post Office Box 20429
Oakland, California 94620

Our books can be found in most bookstores.